SIBO DIET FOR BEGINNERS

1200 Days of Digestive Transformation | Embark on a Journey to Reclaim Gut Health and Enjoy a Life of Comfort and Vitality with the Ultimate Guide to SIBO Management

TALIA HIGGINS

TABLE OF CONTENTS

INTRODUCTION

If you're struggling with persistent gastrointestinal issues and suspect that SIBO may be the root cause, this book is tailored for you. As we journey together towards improved gut health, you will find all the resources necessary to navigate every stage of your SIBO recovery.

In the following chapters, you will learn about the causes and symptoms of SIBO, as well as crucial information on diagnostic procedures and how to interpret test results. You will also be introduced to the core principles of various SIBO diets and gain insight into building a personalized meal plan tailored to your unique needs.

As you progress through the elimination phase of your SIBO diet, this book will provide guidance on foods to avoid, tackling common challenges, and offer delicious meal plans and recipe ideas. Following this critical stage, we focus on reintroducing foods safely into your diet while implementing gut-healing strategies and supplements to promote optimal gut health.

Beyond food choices, this guide also addresses day-to-day challenges such as dining out with dietary restrictions, navigating social gatherings, and traveling while on the SIBO diet. You'll find practical advice on communicating your needs effectively and selecting suitable meals and snacks when away from home.

Emotional eating and stress can significantly impact our health, particularly our gut health. To address these factors, we provide valuable tips for managing emotional eating triggers, adapting mindful eating practices, and implementing stress-reduction techniques designed to support better gut health as part of the healing process.

Family integration is crucial for those following a SIBO diet. You'll discover ways to create satisfying meals that suit everyone's preferences while promoting healthy habits amongst your children.

Finally, this book will help you sustain long-term success in managing SIBO by offering strategies for continuous symptom monitoring and embracing a lifetime of gut-friendly habits. With the knowledge, tools, and support found here, you will reclaim your gut health and enjoy life without the discomfort of SIBO.

CHAPTER 1:
UNDERSTANDING SIBO

Small Intestinal Bacterial Overgrowth (SIBO) is a medical condition characterized by an abnormally high number of bacteria in the small intestine. When these bacteria grow uncontrollably, they disrupt the normal functioning of the gastrointestinal tract and often lead to various symptoms and complications. In this chapter, we will explore the causes, symptoms, diagnosis, and treatment options for SIBO.

Causes of SIBO

Several factors can contribute to the development of SIBO. Some of the most common causes are:

1. Impaired gut motility: A reduction in the movement of food through the digestive system increases the likelihood of bacterial overgrowth.

2. Structural abnormalities: Diverticula or adhesions can result in areas where bacteria can accumulate.

3. Immune system dysfunction: A weakened immune system may be less effective at controlling bacterial growth.

4. Medication use: Prolonged use of certain medications, including acid-blocking drugs (PPIs) and antibiotics, can alter gut microbiome balance.

Identifying Common SIBO Symptoms

To help you identify if you may be experiencing this condition, here are the common symptoms associated with SIBO:

1. Abdominal pain and bloating: One of the most common SIBO symptoms is abdominal discomfort accompanied by a sense of fullness or distention. This bloating may worsen after meals or become persistent throughout the day.

2. Diarrhea: Frequent, loose stools are another typical symptom of SIBO. The excess bacteria in the small intestine can disrupt normal digestion and absorption processes, leading to diarrhea.

3. Constipation: Despite being contradictory to diarrhea, some individuals with SIBO may experience constipation instead. The imbalance of gut bacteria can slow down intestinal motility, resulting in infrequent or difficult bowel movements.

4. Gas and flatulence: Excessive gas production is a common issue related to SIBO. The fermentation of undigested food by the overgrown bacteria often leads to increased flatulence and sometimes foul-smelling gas.

5. Nausea and acid reflux: Nausea and acid reflux can occur due to the disturbance in gastrointestinal functioning caused by SIBO. These symptoms may be more pronounced after consuming certain trigger foods or beverages.

6. Fatigue: Persistent fatigue can accompany SIBO, often as a result of malabsorption of vital nutrients due to impaired digestion.

7. Unexplained weight loss: Weight loss without an obvious cause may signal SIBO, particularly if it coincides with other digestive symptoms listed above.

8. Nutrient deficiencies: In addition to malabsorption causing weight loss and fatigue, it can also result in nutrient deficiencies such as anemia or vitamin deficiencies, which may further exacerbate health problems.

The Impact of SIBO On Gut Health

SIBO can significantly impact gut health in various ways, some of which include:

1. Malabsorption: Excessive bacteria in the small intestine can interfere with proper nutrient absorption. These bacteria consume the essential nutrients meant for our body, leading to vitamin and mineral deficiencies which can cause symptoms such as fatigue, weight loss, and anemia.

2. Intestinal Inflammation: SIBO often leads to inflammation of the small intestine as a result of excessive bacterial growth. This inflammation not only compromises nutrient absorption but also damages the intestinal lining and impairs its functions.

3. Altered Gut Motility: Having an increased number of bacteria in the small intestine can affect gut motility – the coordinated contractions responsible for moving food through the digestive tract. Disruptions in gut motility can further contribute to bacterial overgrowth and lead to symptoms like bloating, abdominal pain, and constipation or diarrhea.

4. Impaired Immune System: The overgrowth of bacteria in the small intestine may disrupt the balance between beneficial and harmful microbes in our gastrointestinal (GI) tract. This imbalance weakens our immune system, making it difficult for our bodies to ward off infections and maintain overall health.

5. Leaky Gut Syndrome: When SIBO causes damage to the intestinal lining, it increases gut permeability, allowing toxins, undigested food particles, and harmful bacteria to leak into the bloodstream leading to a condition known as leaky gut syndrome – which has been linked with various autoimmune disorders and chronic health issues.

6. Mental Health Implications: The gut and brain are closely connected, and any disruptions in gut health can significantly affect mental well-being. SIBO has been linked to psychological symptoms such as anxiety, depression, and brain fog.

CHAPTER 2:
DIAGNOSING SIBO

Accurate diagnosis of SIBO is essential for determining the appropriate treatment plan and improving patient outcomes. This chapter provides an overview of the diagnostic tests available for identifying SIBO.

1. Hydrogen and Methane Breath Test: It is a non-invasive method to detect SIBO. This test measures the levels of hydrogen and methane gases in your breath after consuming a sugar solution (lactulose or glucose). Elevated levels of these gases indicate the excessive bacteria in your small intestine. The breath test involves fasting for 12 hours before taking the test, then consuming the sugar solution and collecting breath samples every 20 minutes for a period of 2-3 hours. This test can provide information about possible bacterial overgrowth and help guide treatment decisions.

2. Small Bowel Aspirate Culture: It involves the collection of a fluid sample from the small intestine during an endoscopy procedure. The fluid is then cultured to identify and quantify bacterial growth. A high concentration of bacteria (usually more than 100,000 CFU/mL) suggests SIBO. This invasive test can provide definitive evidence of bacterial overgrowth but may not be suitable for all patients due to its invasive nature and potential risk for complications.

3. Glucose Breath Test: It is another non-invasive diagnostic tool that uses glucose as its substrate to detect bacterial overgrowth in your small intestine by measuring hydrogen concentrations in your exhale during a series of timed intervals after consumption of glucose solution. High levels of hydrogen signal excessive bacteria in the small intestine.

4. Full-Length GI Transit Time Test: This test is designed to determine the time it takes for food to pass through the gastrointestinal tract, which can provide insight into potential motility issues contributing to SIBO. Patients swallow a wireless capsule that records its position as it moves through the GI system, and this data is used to calculate transit times. Prolonged transit times may indicate an increased risk of SIBO development due to slowed gastrointestinal motility.

5. Serum Tests: Blood tests can be beneficial in identifying possible underlying conditions or deficiencies that may be contributing factors to the development of SIBO. Some of these tests include serum vitamin B12 levels, iron levels, and serum folate levels. Patients with SIBO often exhibit deficiencies in these nutrients due to malabsorption caused by excessive bacterial growth.

6. Exclusionary Diagnostics: Exclusionary diagnostics involve ruling out other potential causes for a patient's symptoms before diagnosing SIBO. These tests can include imaging studies (e.g., CT scan or

MRI), endoscopy and biopsy procedures, and assessment for conditions like celiac disease, inflammatory bowel disease, and pancreatic insufficiency.

Interpreting SIBO Test Results

Diagnosing SIBO is crucial for proper treatment and management of the condition. The most widely used method for diagnosing SIBO is the hydrogen and methane breath test. This section will focus on interpreting the results of this test to better understand and manage SIBO.

The hydrogen and methane breath test measures the amount of hydrogen (H2) and methane (CH4) gases produced by bacteria in the small intestine. These gases are then exhaled and can be detected through a breath sample. The test begins with an individual fasting overnight and then consuming a solution containing a specific type of sugar (such as lactulose or glucose). Over the next few hours, breath samples are collected at regular intervals, usually every 15-20 minutes.

The rationale behind this test is that when certain types of bacteria break down carbohydrates in the small intestine, they produce H2 and CH4 as byproducts. These gases are not produced by human cells; therefore, elevated levels indicate bacterial overgrowth. Here's how to interpret SIBO test results based on hydrogen and methane levels:

1. Hydrogen-Dominant SIBO: If an individual's breath sample shows a significant increase in hydrogen levels (>20 parts per million) within 90-120 minutes after ingesting the sugar solution, it suggests hydrogen-dominant SIBO. Bacteria that produce hydrogen gas are usually anaerobic or facultative anaerobic bacteria.

2. Methane-Dominant SIBO: A significant increase in methane levels (>10 parts per million) within 90-120 minutes after ingesting the sugar solution indicates methane-dominant SIBO. Bacteria that produce methane are called methanogens and belong to the archaea domain.

3. Mixed SIBO: Some individuals may show an increase in both hydrogen and methane levels in their breath samples. This is indicative of mixed-type SIBO, where both types of bacteria are present in the small intestine.

4. Hydrogen Sulfide SIBO: In some cases, neither hydrogen nor methane levels may increase during the test. Instead, the individual's symptoms may be due to hydrogen sulfide (H2S) producing bacteria. Unfortunately, current breath testing methods cannot accurately detect H2S; however, researchers are currently working on developing new testing methods for hydrogen sulfide SIBO.

It is essential to consider that breath test results alone may not provide a definitive diagnosis of SIBO. False positives can occur due to factors such as improper test preparation or incorrect interpretation of results by laboratory personnel. Additionally, false negatives are also possible when bacterial overgrowth occurs deeper in the small intestine or if specific gas-producing bacteria are not present.

Consulting with Healthcare Professionals

Proper diagnosis and treatment of SIBO rely on consulting with healthcare professionals experienced in diagnosing and managing gastrointestinal disorders. When consulting with medical professionals, it's essential to provide comprehensive information regarding your medical history and all symptoms experienced to ensure an accurate diagnosis.

Additionally, healthcare professionals may recommend a combination of treatment options, such as dietary changes, antimicrobial therapy, or probiotics, depending on the severity and underlying causes of SIBO. Regular follow-up with healthcare professionals is crucial for monitoring progress and adjusting the treatment plan as needed.

CHAPTER 3:
SIBO DIET BASICS

The SIBO diet aims to restore balance in the digestive system by providing nutrient-dense, easily digestible foods while minimizing those that contribute to bacterial overgrowth. This chapter provides an in-depth overview of the SIBO diet, its principles, benefits, and helpful tips for those considering adopting this diet to manage their digestive issues.

The SIBO diet revolves around specific principles to promote gut health by creating an unfavorable environment for harmful bacteria. It consists of three main components:

1. Restricted carbohydrate intake: A key principle in managing bacterial overgrowth is reducing carbohydrates that bacteria feed on. Excessive carbohydrates can trigger bacterial fermentation, leading to gas production and worsening of symptoms. The SIBO diet includes complex carbohydrates such as non-starchy vegetables and excludes simple sugars and starchy vegetables like grains, potatoes, and legumes.

2. Emphasis on low FODMAP foods: FODMAPs are short-chain carbohydrates that can be poorly absorbed by some people leading to abdominal pain and bloating. Low FODMAP foods are easier to digest and reduce symptoms associated with bacterial overgrowth. The SIBO diet encourages consuming low FODMAP vegetables like leafy greens, chives, bell peppers, carrots, zucchini, tomatoes, cucumber, and green beans.

3. Optimal distribution of meals: To manage SIBO effectively; timing meal consumption is crucial. The goal is not only what you eat but when you eat it. The SIBO diet emphasizes three main meals per day without snacking between them—which allows time for your gastrointestinal system to efficiently digest ingested food, thereby limiting bacterial fermentation.

The benefits of adopting a SIBO diet are multifaceted. While the primary goal is to manage bacterial overgrowth, many other positive effects are observed in those following this nutrition plan:

1. Improved digestion: By removing trigger foods and including easy-to-digest options, the SIBO diet reduces symptoms related to bacterial overgrowth. This leads to a decrease in bloating, gas, diarrhea, or constipation.

2. Reduced inflammation: As the SIBO diet supports an overall healthy digestive system, it consequently helps reduce inflammation associated with gastrointestinal issues. Lowering inflammation can lead to better overall gut function and reduced pain or discomfort.

3. Enhanced nutrient absorption: A significant challenge with SIBO is the compromised absorption of nutrients due to bacteria overgrowth in the small intestine. The SIBO diet aids in improving nutrient absorption by providing easily digestible foods that minimize inflammation and enhance gut function.

4. Increased energy levels: By following well-balanced, nutrient-dense diet plan rich in low FODMAP foods and reducing reliance on carbohydrates as an energy source, individuals may notice increased energy levels as their body adapts to alternative energy sources like proteins and fats.

5. Weight management: Although not designed as a weight management plan, it's common for individuals with SIBO to experience weight fluctuations due to digestive issues and malnutrition before starting this diet. By consuming nutrient-dense foods that support a healthy gut flora and not relying on snacking between meals, the SIBO diet can contribute to effective weight management for those who need it.

It's also worth mentioning that one should consider consulting with a healthcare professional or registered dietitian before starting any new dietary approach. A tailored approach based on individual needs often proves most successful when handling complex digestive issues such as SIBO.

With more people affected each day by digestive issues like bloating, diarrhea, and abdominal pain, the significance of the SIBO diet should not be overlooked. By introducing this dietary approach, managing symptoms becomes significantly more comfortable as it targets the root cause of bacterial overgrowth in the small intestine. Furthermore, adhering to the principles mentioned above can lead to significant improvements in not just gut health but overall well-being.

Types of SIBO Diets and Their Benefits

There are several different types of SIBO diets that focus on eliminating specific foods to help alleviate symptoms and reduce bacterial growth. Let's explore four popular SIBO diets and their benefits:

1. Low FODMAP Diet: The Low FODMAP (Fermentable Oligosaccharides, Disaccharides, Monosaccharides and Polyols) diet is perhaps the most well-known diet for managing SIBO. The main principle behind this diet is to minimize the consumption of fermentable carbohydrates that serve as food for the overgrown bacteria in the small intestine.

FODMAPs are present in wheat, onions, garlic, beans and legumes, dairy products, fruits such as apples, pears and peaches, and certain vegetables like broccoli, cauliflower and cabbage.

A Low FODMAP diet consists of three phases: elimination, reintroduction and personalization. During the elimination phase, all high-FODMAP foods are avoided for 4-6 weeks. After that comes the reintroduction phase where individuals systematically test their tolerance to varying levels of FODMAPs by slowly reintroducing them into their diet. The last phase is personalization adapting a long-term eating plan based on individual tolerance levels.

Benefits:

- [ ] Reduction in digestive symptoms such as bloating and abdominal pain
- [ ] Improved bowel function
- [ ] Better overall digestive health

2. Specific Carbohydrate Diet (SCD): It aims to restore the balance of gut bacteria by restricting complex carbohydrates. On this diet plan, monosaccharides or simple sugars are allowed, while disaccharides and polysaccharides such as lactose, sucrose, and maltose are avoided.

The SCD diet allows most fruits, vegetables, nuts, meat, fish, and eggs. Processed and packaged foods are generally off-limits. This approach can be beneficial for those with SIBO but may require further adjustments based on individual needs.

Benefits:

- [ ] Improvement in digestive symptoms
- [ ] Repletion of micronutrients often depleted in SIBO sufferers

3. Gut and Psychology Syndrome (GAPS) Diet: It is designed to heal the gut lining, restore gut flora balance, and improve neurological health. It is a more restrictive dietary approach that focuses on homemade bone broth, fermented foods, and organic animal-based proteins.

The GAPS diet comprises three main stages: the introduction stage with a limited food selection focusing on broths and cooked vegetables; the full GAPS stage wherein more variety is introduced gradually; and the reintroduction stage when foods not allowed in previous stages are tested for tolerance.

Benefits:

- [ ] Improves overall gut health
- [ ] Enhances immune system functioning
- [ ] Aids in neurological function improvement

4. SIBO Bi-phasic Diet: It is a two-phase dietary plan developed by Dr. Nirala Jacobi that combines elements from both Low FODMAP and SCD diets. The first phase is designed to calm the symptoms by limiting specific foods for 4-6 weeks; the second phase progressively reintroduces higher-FODMAP foods while remaining low-starch.

Benefits:

- [ ] Effectively manages SIBO symptoms
- [ ] Provides a structured approach to reintroducing foods
- [ ] Tailored specifically for individuals with SIBO

Each SIBO diet has its unique benefits, and the choice depends on personal preference, dietary needs, and the severity of the condition. Consulting a healthcare professional or nutritionist is crucial when deciding on the appropriate diet plan for managing SIBO symptoms. With the right guidance, individuals can find relief and improve their overall digestive health through specific dietary modifications.

Building A Personalized SIBO Meal Plan

A personalized SIBO meal plan not only takes into account individual food preferences but also helps to lower the risk of symptom flare-ups. Follow these steps to create a tailored meal plan that can help manage SIBO:

1. Consult a Nutrition Professional: Before attempting to create a meal plan on your own, consult with a nutritionist or registered dietitian who has experience working with SIBO patients. These professionals can help identify triggers and recommend dietary modifications based on individual needs.

2. Identify Sensitive Foods: Some common food types can exacerbate SIBO symptoms—for example, high FODMAP foods may increase bacterial growth in the small intestine. With the guidance of a healthcare professional, identify any foods that worsen symptoms and eliminate them from your diet temporarily.

3. Choose Low FODMAP Foods: Initially, opt for low FODMAP foods to nourish your body without providing substrates for unwanted bacterial growth. Examples include lean meats, fish, eggs, non-dairy milk alternatives (e.g., almond milk), gluten-free grains (e.g., quinoa and rice), and certain fruits and vegetables (e.g., blueberries and carrots).

4. Reintroduce Foods Gradually: After a period of following the low FODMAP diet—typically 6-8 weeks—begin reintroducing higher FODMAP foods one at a time while keeping track of any symptom changes. This process helps to identify specific ingredients that may be contributing to SIBO symptoms.

5. Hydration: Staying well-hydrated throughout the day with water, herbal teas, and other non-caffeinated beverages is essential for proper digestion and overall wellbeing. Aim for at least 2-3 liters of fluid per day.

6. Incorporate Natural Antimicrobials: Some natural compounds may help reduce bacterial overgrowth in people with SIBO. Consider adding foods with antimicrobial properties such as coconut oil, garlic, ginger, oregano, and thyme to your meal plan.

7. Follow a Consistent Eating Schedule: Establishing a regular eating schedule can help regulate the digestive system. Aim to eat three balanced meals a day, along with snacks as needed. Try not to skip meals or eat erratically which can worsen SIBO symptoms.

8. Mindful Eating Practices: Practicing mindful eating habits can help aid in digestion and decrease stress-related stomach issues. Chew your food thoroughly and eat slowly, allowing sufficient time for digestion before consuming more food.

9. Monitor Nutrient Intake: People with SIBO may experience poor nutrient absorption due to imbalances in their gut flora. Ensuring that you are getting essential nutrients from your diet is vital for overall health and wellness. Consider working with a healthcare professional to monitor macronutrients (protein, carbohydrates, fats) and micronutrients (vitamins and minerals) intake levels.

10. Adapt the Meal Plan as Needed: Since SIBO symptoms can change over time or improve with treatment, regularly re-evaluate your meal plan in collaboration with your healthcare provider to ensure it addresses your current needs and preferences appropriately.

Creating a personalized SIBO meal plan requires patience, persistence, and attention to the individual's unique needs, preferences, and tolerances. It's crucial to work closely with healthcare professionals throughout this process to optimize dietary strategies, ensuring a balanced and satisfying meal plan that addresses symptoms and supports overall health and well-being.

CHAPTER 4:
NAVIGATING THE
ELIMINATION PHASE

The elimination phase of the SIBO diet is a crucial step in managing symptoms and restoring gastrointestinal balance. This phase involves identifying and removing trigger foods that contribute to symptoms such as bloating, gas, diarrhea, constipation, and abdominal pain. Although this phase can be challenging, understanding its importance and following a few key strategies can make the process smoother and more effective.

The primary goal of the elimination phase in the SIBO diet is to starve the overgrown bacteria in the small intestine by cutting off their food sources, i.e., fermentable carbohydrates. These are found in numerous foods, including some fruits, vegetables, grains, legumes, dairy products and certain sugars. By eliminating these potential triggers from your diet for a specified period (usually 4-6 weeks), you give your gut a chance to heal while also learning which specific foods exacerbate your symptoms.

Strategies for Navigating the Elimination Phase

1. Start with a comprehensive food list: Work with a healthcare practitioner or nutritionist experienced in SIBO diets to provide you with an extensive list of allowed and disallowed foods during this phase. This essential guide will be your primary resource and help keep you on track as you make dietary adjustments.

2. Plan and prepare meals: With numerous restrictions during the elimination phase, planning meals in advance can help save time, reduce stress, and minimize food-related slip-ups. Dedicate some time each week to plan your meals based on allowed SIBO-friendly ingredients. Consider cooking larger portions that can be stored for easy reheating or repurposing throughout the week.

3. Gradually introduce new foods: As you eliminate certain types of carbohydrates from your diet during this phase, aim to slowly reintroduce new foods into your meal plan one at a time. This cautious reintroduction allows you to observe any potential reactions or symptoms and pinpoint the specific foods causing you issues.

4. Keep a food diary: Track your meals, snacks and symptoms throughout the elimination phase. By keeping a detailed account of what you're consuming and any subsequent reactions, you can identify potential trigger foods more accurately. This information will be invaluable when working with your healthcare practitioner to personalize your SIBO diet.

5. Stay hydrated and nourished: While the focus may be on eliminating certain foods, it's equally essential to ensure you're meeting your daily nutritional needs. Drink plenty of water, consume a variety of allowed nutrient-dense foods, choose lean protein sources and prioritize gut-healing nutrients such as bone broth, collagen peptides, or omega-3 fatty acids from wild-caught fish or fish oil supplements.

6. Enlist support: Navigating a restrictive diet like the SIBO elimination phase can feel isolating at times. Don't hesitate to seek support from both professionals and peers, whether it's finding others through online forums, local support groups or even connecting with friends who have undergone similar dietary changes.

7. Embrace patience and self-compassion: Remember that healing your gut is neither a linear nor speedy process. It is normal to experience ups and downs during the elimination phase, so practice patience and self-compassion during this challenging time.

Once your symptoms have significantly improved, work with your healthcare practitioner to determine when it's appropriate to move from the elimination phase into the reintroduction phase. In this subsequent stage, previously eliminated foods are gradually added back in order to assess your tolerance levels and tailor a long-term nutrition plan specific to your individual needs.

Foods To Avoid During the Elimination Phase

Here are some of the main foods you should avoid during this phase.

1. High-FODMAP Foods: These are a group of carbohydrates that can be challenging to digest and often ferment in the gut. These carbs can exacerbate SIBO symptoms by providing a food source for bacteria to thrive. Common high-FODMAP foods to avoid during the Elimination Phase include:

- ☐ Fructose: Honey, apples, pears, watermelon
- ☐ Lactose: Milk, yogurt, ice cream
- ☐ Fructans: Wheat-based products like bread, pasta, various vegetables (e.g., garlic and onion)
- ☐ Galactans: Legumes like beans, lentils, soy

2. Sugary Foods: Sugar feeds the overgrown bacteria in the small intestine and can worsen SIBO symptoms. Stay clear of:

- ☐ Added sugars: Found in soft drinks, candy, baked goods
- ☐ Natural sugars (with moderation): Fruit juices and dried fruits
- ☐ Artificial sweeteners: Sorbitol and Mannitol

3. Alcohol: Alcohol can impair gut motility and have a negative impact on beneficial gut bacteria. It also contains sugars that feed harmful bacteria. It is best to avoid alcohol entirely during the Elimination Phase.

4. Dairy Products: Lactose is found in dairy products, which can be difficult to digest and end up feeding the bacteria in the small intestine. Some alternatives include lactose-free dairy products or non-dairy substitutes.

5. Processed and Refined Foods: Processed foods often contain added sugar, unhealthy fats, and artificial ingredients that may cause bloating, gas, and negative effects on beneficial gut bacteria. During the Elimination Phase, avoid these types of foods:

- ☐ Canned and packaged foods
- ☐ Refined grains (e.g., white rice, white bread)
- ☐ Instant meals
- ☐ Fast food

6. Complex Carbohydrates: Foods high in complex carbohydrates like grains, starchy vegetables, and legumes should be limited as they provide fuel for bacteria to grow. Some examples of these foods to avoid are:

- ☐ Potatoes
- ☐ Corn
- ☐ Pasta
- ☐ Beans

7. Cruciferous Vegetables: While these vegetables are healthy and nutritious, they can cause gas and bloating in some individuals due to their high fiber content, especially during the Elimination Phase of a SIBO Diet. Examples of cruciferous vegetables to limit or avoid are:

- ☐ Broccoli
- ☐ Cauliflower
- ☐ Brussels sprouts
- ☐ Cabbage

8. Certain Nuts and Seeds: Nuts and seeds that are high in carbohydrates can contribute to bacterial overgrowth. However, not all nuts and seeds need to be avoided — only those with higher carbohydrate content like cashews and pistachios should be excluded during the Elimination Phase.

9. Carbonated Beverages: These drinks consist of bubbles flavored with sugar or artificial sweeteners, making this both a no-go for your gut health and SIBO diet plan.

Overcoming Common Challenges During the Elimination Phase

One of the essential components of the SIBO diet is the elimination phase, which lasts anywhere between 2-6 weeks. During this phase, it is crucial to avoid highly fermentable foods to starve the bacteria in the small intestine. However, several challenges can arise during this phase, making it difficult for people to stick to their new meal plan. Here are some tips for overcoming these common obstacles.

1. Cravings and temptations: One of the biggest challenges during the elimination phase is managing cravings and resisting temptations. As you eliminate certain foods from your diet, it's normal to crave them even more. To cope with these cravings:

- Pre-plan your meals to ensure you have delicious and satisfying options available that conform to your dietary restrictions.
- Keep healthy snacks on hand which align with the SIBO elimination phase. Some examples include nuts, seeds, and low-sugar fruits.
- Drink plenty of water throughout the day; staying hydrated can help curb hunger pangs.
- Maintain a food diary to gain insight into your eating patterns and identify triggers that may lead to cravings.

2. Social situations: Eating out or attending social gatherings can prove difficult when you're adhering to specific dietary guidelines. To overcome this challenge:

- Research restaurants beforehand and find out if they offer dishes that are suitable for your dietary requirements.
- Don't hesitate to communicate your dietary needs with restaurant staff so they can guide you in choosing appropriate menu options.
- If you're attending a social gathering, bring a SIBO friendly dish. Not only will you have something safe to eat, but it also allows others to sample your healthy cuisine.

3. Food preparation and planning: Cooking and meal planning can be daunting tasks when starting a new diet. To make it easier:

- Spend some time each week meal prepping. Batch cook and store meals in the refrigerator or freezer for later use.
- Keep a list of your favorite recipes handy so that you can easily reference them while shopping or cooking.
- Invest in an instant pot, slow cooker, or air fryer. These kitchen gadgets can simplify meal preparation and reduce cooking time.
- Schedule time for grocery shopping and prioritize stores that stock fresh produce and high-quality ingredients.

4. Reintroducing foods: One of the most significant challenges of the elimination phase is reintroducing foods after the initial weeks of restriction. This process can be tricky, as missteps may lead to flare-ups of your symptoms. Here are some tips for tackling this challenge:

☐ Gradually reintroduce one food at a time, allowing your body to adjust.

☐ Monitor your symptoms closely during reintroductions; keep track of any adverse reactions in your food diary.

☐ Consult with a dietitian or healthcare professional for guidance on safe reintroduction practices.

5. Maintaining motivation and staying on track: Staying motivated during the elimination phase can be challenging, but it's essential to stay committed to experiencing relief from SIBO symptoms. To stay motivated:

☐ Track your progress by noting improvements in your symptoms and overall well-being in your food diary.

☐ Keep communication open with your healthcare provider for support and guidance throughout the process.

☐ Reach out to online forums or local support groups where you can connect with others going through similar experiences.

6. Nutrient deficiencies: As the elimination phase of the SIBO diet requires cutting out specific foods, it's possible to face nutrient deficiencies. To avoid this issue:

☐ Eat a diverse range of allowable foods that provide essential vitamins and minerals.

☐ Consult with your healthcare professional or dietitian to determine if supplementation is necessary for your specific needs.

By foreseeing challenges and being prepared with strategies for overcoming them, you'll be better equipped to navigate the elimination phase of the SIBO diet successfully. Stay motivated, educate yourself about food options, and seek guidance from professionals as needed.

Sample Meal Plans
and
Recipe Ideas

SIBO diet aims to alleviate gastrointestinal symptoms by reducing the number of bacteria in the small intestine. It's essential to plan meals that can help achieve this goal while also providing adequate nutrition. Below are three meal plans designed for each benefit, along with a recipe example for each meal.

Meal Plan 1:

☐ *Breakfast:* Gluten-free oatmeal with berries and almonds
☐ *Lunch:* Grilled chicken salad with mixed greens, cucumbers, red bell peppers, and vinaigrette dressing
☐ *Dinner:* Baked salmon with steamed green beans and quinoa

NOTES

_____

_____

_____

Recipe Example
GRILLED CHICKEN SALAD

Preparation time: 10 minutes
Cooking time: 15 minutes
Servings: 2

Ingredients:

- ☐ Half pound grilled chicken breast
- ☐ Four cups mixed greens
- ☐ Half cucumber, sliced
- ☐ Half red bell pepper, sliced

Vinaigrette Dressing:

- ☐ Two tbsp olive oil
- ☐ One tbsp apple cider vinegar
- ☐ Salt & pepper, as required

Directions:

1. Grill the chicken breast until fully cooked. Put aside.
2. Mix greens, cucumber, plus bell pepper slices in your big container. Slice the grilled chicken breast, then add it to your salad.
3. In your small container, whisk oil, vinegar, salt plus pepper. Drizzle it on salad, then toss gently. Serve.

Nutritional Values (per serving): *Calories: 424; Carbs: 15g; Fat: 26g; Protein: 35g; Fiber: 5g*

NOTES

_____

_____

_____

Meal Plan 2:

- [ ] *Breakfast:* Greek yogurt with blueberries, chia seeds, and cinnamon
- [ ] *Lunch:* Spinach and goat cheese-stuffed chicken breast with a side of steamed broccoli
- [ ] *Dinner:* Pan-seared shrimp with zucchini noodles and cherry tomatoes

NOTES

_____

_____

_____

Recipe Example
GREEK YOGURT BREAKFAST BOWL

Preparation time: 5 minutes
Cooking time: 0 minutes
Servings: 1

Ingredients:

- [ ] One cup Greek yogurt (full-fat or low-fat)
- [ ] Half cup fresh blueberries
- [ ] One tbsp chia seeds
- [ ] A pinch of cinnamon

Directions:

1. Place the Greek yogurt in your bowl. Add fresh blueberries on top, then sprinkle chia seeds.
2. Finish with a pinch of cinnamon. Stir gently before consuming.

Nutritional Values (per serving): *Calories: 303; Carbs: 29g; Fat: 9g; Protein: 25g; Fiber: 7g*

NOTES

_____

_____

_____

Meal Plan 3:

- [ ] *Breakfast:* Two-egg vegetable omelet with spinach, bell peppers, and feta cheese
- [ ] *Lunch:* Turkey lettuce wraps with avocado, red onion, and mustard sauce
- [ ] *Dinner:* Lemon herb roast chicken with carrots and green beans

NOTES

_____

_____

_____

Recipe Example

TURKEY LETTUCE WRAPS

Preparation time: 10 minutes
Cooking time: 0 minutes
Servings: 2

Ingredients:

- ☐ Four iceberg lettuce leaves
- ☐ Half pound sliced turkey breast
- ☐ One small avocado, sliced
- ☐ Quarter red onion, thinly sliced
- ☐ Two tbsp mustard sauce

Directions:

1. Lay out the iceberg lettuce leaves on your clean surface. Divide turkey breast evenly among your lettuce leaves. Top each wrap with avocado slices and red onion.
2. Drizzle mustard sauce over each wrap, then fold the lettuce leaves to enclose the fillings.

Nutritional Values (per serving): *Calories: 225; Carbs: 6g; Fat: 12g; Protein: 24g; Fiber: 3g*

NOTES

_____

_____

_____

CHAPTER 5:
REINTRODUCING FOODS
AND HEALING THE GUT

Treating SIBO often involves the use of antibiotics and dietary modifications. After successful treatment with antibiotics, it is crucial to reintroduce foods gradually in order to minimize symptoms and maintain a healthy gut environment.

The first step in gradually reintroducing foods into the diet for SIBO is understanding which foods can be safely added back without aggravating symptoms or contributing to potential bad bacteria overgrowth. The following guidelines are helpful when beginning the process of reintroducing foods:

1. Start with a Low-FODMAP diet: The Low-FODMAP diet is often recommended for individuals with SIBO because it minimizes the intake of certain types of carbohydrates that are poorly absorbed by the small intestine and can lead to bacterial overgrowth. Gradually introducing low-FODMAP foods such as lean proteins, low-lactose dairy, and non-dense complex carbohydrates will help your digestive system adapt while minimizing the likelihood of triggering symptoms.

2. Reintroduce one food at a time: To gauge your body's reaction to specific foods, introduce one new food every three days. This will allow you to identify any potential food triggers that may worsen your SIBO symptoms without overwhelming your gut. Keep a journal to track which foods you have introduced and any symptoms or reactions experienced after consuming them.

3. Begin with smaller portions: As you reintroduce each new food, start with a small portion size and see how your body reacts Initially, small servings can help minimize potential gut distress caused by larger quantities of high-FODMAP foods or those that are harder to digest.

4. Prioritize nutrient-dense foods: Maintaining a balanced diet is essential for overall health and wellbeing. Focus on reintroducing nutrient-dense foods that provide essential vitamins, minerals, and nutrients to support your body's healing process and promote overall gut health.

5. Gradually increase portion sizes: Once you have successfully reintroduced a food without causing any adverse reaction or symptoms, you can start to increase the portion size. However, it is important to monitor your body's response during this process to ensure that you do not overwhelm your gut with too much food at once.

6. Reintroduce probiotic-rich foods: After successfully reintroducing low-FODMAP foods and ensuring there are no adverse reactions, you can begin slowly integrating fermented foods such as sauerkraut, kimchi, yogurt, and kefir into the diet. These probiotic-rich foods help promote a diverse gut microbiome by introducing beneficial bacteria that aid in digestion and overall gut health.

7. Avoid foods that tend to exacerbate SIBO symptoms: Certain carbohydrates such as refined grains, sugars, and high-fructose corn syrup can contribute to bacterial overgrowth in the small intestine. It is advisable to continue avoiding these types of foods even after your initial treatment for SIBO is complete.

8. Listen to your body: Throughout this entire process, it is essential to be mindful of how specific foods affect your body and make adjustments accordingly. If a certain food triggers symptoms or causes discomfort, remove it from the diet temporarily and try again after a few weeks when your gut has had more time to heal.

9. Consult with a healthcare professional: If you are unsure about how best to reintroduce foods into your diet following SIBO treatment or experience significant discomfort during the process, consult with a healthcare professional experienced in treating digestive disorders. They can offer guidance on the best approach for gradual reintroduction tailored to your specific needs.

Gut-Healing Strategies and Supplements for SIBO

In order to combat SIBO and promote gut healing, it is important to incorporate strategies and supplements that can help restore balance to the gut flora. Here are some gut-healing strategies and supplements that may be beneficial for SIBO:

1. Diet Modification: One of the primary ways to promote gut healing and manage SIBO is through dietary changes. The Low FODMAP diet has been shown to be effective in reducing symptoms related to SIBO. This diet limits the consumption of fermentable carbohydrates which are known to feed bad bacteria in the gut, therefore helping curb the growth of these bacteria.

Some foods that can be included in a low FODMAP diet are lean meats, fish, eggs, certain fruits and vegetables such as bananas, blueberries, carrots, and bell peppers, as well as gluten-free grains like rice and quinoa.

2. Probiotics: Probiotics contain beneficial microorganisms that support a healthy gut environment. Research suggests that taking probiotics may assist in reducing bacterial overgrowth and subsequently alleviating symptoms associated with SIBO. Look for probiotics that contain a mixture of strains like Lactobacillus and Bifidobacterium that have been proven to be effective.

3. Digestive Enzymes: Digestive enzymes play an essential role in breaking down food into smaller particles for better absorption by the body. By supplementing with digestive enzymes, individuals with SIBO may improve digestion, reduce bloating and gas while creating a less favorable environment for harmful bacteria thriving in undigested food particles.

4. Herbal Antibiotics: Herbal antibiotics can offer a natural alternative to conventional antibiotics for the treatment of SIBO. Some commonly used herbal antibiotics include oregano oil, berberine, and allicin (derived from garlic). These herbs have antimicrobial properties that target unwanted bacteria without disrupting the beneficial gut flora like prescription antibiotics may do.

5. L-Glutamine: It is an amino acid that helps maintain the integrity of the gut lining and supports its repair process. It is especially helpful for individuals with SIBO, as it assists in reducing inflammation and preventing the leakage of harmful substances into the bloodstream through a compromised gut barrier.

6. Zinc-carnosine: Zinc-carnosine is a combination of the essential mineral zinc and an amino acid called carnosine. This compound promotes gut healing by stabilizing the gut lining, exhibiting antioxidant properties, and providing anti-inflammatory effects.

7. Prebiotics: Prebiotics are non-digestible fibers that act as food for beneficial gut bacteria. Although they should be introduced carefully in individuals with SIBO, they can play an essential role in promoting the growth of good bacteria once bacterial overgrowth has been addressed.

8. Vitamin D: Vitamin D is a fat-soluble vitamin crucial for overall health and proper immune function. Research shows that increased vitamin D levels are associated with a healthier balance of gut bacteria. As such, supplementing with vitamin D can help support the recovery of a balanced gut environment in individuals with SIBO.

9. Omega-3 fatty acids: Omega-3 fatty acids have been shown to improve gut health due to their anti-inflammatory properties. They can be found in foods like fatty fish, algae, flaxseeds, chia seeds, or taken as supplements via fish oil or algae-derived capsules.

10. Fiber Supplements: Fiber supplements should be introduced cautiously when dealing with SIBO since some fiber sources may exacerbate symptoms. However, once SIBO is resolved, incorporating soluble fibers like psyllium or partially hydrolyzed guar gum may help prevent relapses by maintaining a strong and balanced gut flora.

Tips For Maintaining a Balanced Gut Microbiome for SIBO

There are several lifestyle modifications and dietary changes that can help maintain a balanced gut microbiome to prevent SIBO. Here are some tips to promote a healthy gut environment:

1. Incorporate Probiotics into Your Diet: They are beneficial bacteria that support a healthy balance of gut microbiota. Consuming probiotic-rich foods regularly can help maintain the balance of good and bad bacteria in the gut ecosystem.

2. Limit the Intake of Sugars and Refined Carbohydrates: Sugars and refined carbohydrates can contribute to bacterial overgrowth in the small intestine when consumed in excess. Reducing your intake of these foods can help prevent SIBO by promoting a balanced gut microbiome. Opt for healthier, complex carbohydrates like whole grains, beans, legumes, vegetables, and fruits.

3. Eat More Fiber-Rich Foods: A diet rich in fiber can help regulate digestion by promoting the growth of beneficial gut bacteria while inhibiting harmful ones from proliferating. Foods high in soluble fiber such as oats, psyllium husk, chia seeds, flaxseeds, barley, and apples can be particularly helpful in preventing SIBO due to their prebiotic properties.

4. Stay Hydrated: Drinking sufficient water is crucial for maintaining optimal digestive function and keeping your gut microbiome healthy. Adequate hydration helps support bowel movements while flushing out waste and toxins, keeping the gut ecosystem in check. Drink eight glasses of water daily and increase your intake during periods of increased activity or hot weather.

5. Exercise Regularly: Regular exercise supports a healthy and diverse gut microbiome by promoting bowel movements, stimulating the production of digestive enzymes, and reducing inflammation. Aim for 30 minutes moderate-intensity exercise such as walking, swimming, or cycling daily.

6. Manage Stress Effectively: Chronic stress can negatively impact your gut microbiome by decreasing the diversity of beneficial bacteria and increasing intestinal permeability. Practice stress-reduction techniques like mindfulness meditation, yoga, deep breathing exercises, or other relaxation methods to help maintain a balanced gut environment.

7. Avoid Overusing Antibiotics: While antibiotics can be life-saving medications, overusing them can lead to an imbalance in your gut microflora as they kill off beneficial bacteria alongside harmful ones. If you must take antibiotics, speak with your doctor about supplementing with probiotics to restore your gut's bacterial balance.

8. Limit Alcohol Consumption: Excessive alcohol intake can disrupt gut function by killing off essential bacteria and promoting intestinal inflammation. Limit alcohol consumption or eliminate it altogether to help support a healthy and diverse gut microbial community.

9. Adopt a Mediterranean Diet: The Mediterranean diet is packed with nutrient-dense foods that promote optimal gut health, such as whole grains, fruits, vegetables, nuts, seeds, legumes, lean proteins, fish, and olive oil. Its emphasis on plant-based foods makes this dietary pattern particularly beneficial for supporting a balanced gut microbiome.

10. Get Enough Sleep: Getting enough sleep is crucial for maintaining overall health and supporting the proper function of the digestive system. Aim for seven to nine hours of quality sleep nightly to give your body sufficient time for repair and regeneration.

CHAPTER 6:
MEAL PLANNING AND PREP

Following a specific diet and incorporating meal planning techniques can help alleviate the discomfort caused by SIBO. Here are some time-saving meal planning tips that will make your life easier when dealing with this condition.

1. Plan ahead: Setting aside time at the beginning of each week to plan out your meals can save you time in the long run. It will help you avoid last-minute stress and ensure that you have all the necessary ingredients for your meals. Make a list of all the recipes you want to try during the week, and create a shopping list based on those recipes.

2. Batch cooking: Preparing large portions of food at once is a great way to save time and effort in the kitchen. Choose recipes that are easy to scale up, and store leftovers properly for later use throughout the week. Some great meal options for batch cooking include soups, stews, casseroles, and roasted vegetables.

3. Use a slow cooker or instant pot: Both slow cookers and instant pots are amazing tools to have in every kitchen as they require minimal effort and allow you to create delicious dishes packed with flavor. Simply add all your ingredients, set it to cook, and come back later to find a delicious meal ready for you.

4. Prioritize simplicity: The simpler your meals are, the less time-consuming they will be to prepare and cook. Focus on recipes with fewer ingredients or with easy-to-prepare components. You can also save time by using pre-cut vegetables or pre-cooked grains or pasta.

5. Embrace repetition: Meal planning becomes much more straightforward when you stick to a few go-to dishes that you know are SIBO-friendly and enjoyable. Incorporating these recipes into your regular meal rotation will save you time and effort in the long run. Look for creative ways to vary the same basic dish, such as swapping out different vegetables or using different proteins.

6. Fill your pantry with SIBO-friendly staples: Stock up on ingredients that are suitable for a SIBO diet, and you will never be caught off guard when preparing a meal. Some essential items to have on hand include gluten-free grains like quinoa or rice, lean proteins, low-FODMAP vegetables and fruits, and healthy fat sources like olive oil or coconut oil.

7. Prep ingredients beforehand: Chopping and preparing ingredients can be time-consuming, so consider prepping them ahead of time. This can be done on weekends or whenever you have free time. Store them in an organized way in the fridge or freezer, so they're ready to use when required.

8. Utilize leftovers: Leftovers are a lifesaver when it comes to meal planning for SIBO. Re-purpose them into new dishes, such as turning leftover grilled chicken into a salad or stir-fry, or use leftovers to make delicious wraps and sandwiches. Ensure proper storage so that food stays fresh for longer.

9. Make double-duty meals: Choose recipes that can easily be transformed into different meals throughout the week. For example, grill extra chicken during dinner to use in salads, wraps, or stir-fries later in the week.

10. Create a meal planning system: Whether you prefer digital calendars or traditional pen and paper methods, establish a system for tracking your meal plans. This will help you stay organized and make it easier to choose meals each week.

By incorporating these time-saving meal planning techniques into your routine, managing a SIBO diet will become more manageable and enjoyable. With a little organization and preparation, eating delicious meals that suit your dietary restrictions is entirely possible.

Batch Cooking
and
Freezer-Friendly Recipes

Batch cooking is an excellent way to prepare meals ahead of time, saving you both time and effort in the kitchen. This becomes especially important when dealing with SIBO, as it can be difficult to find suitable recipes. In this section, we will share two SIBO-friendly, freezer-friendly recipes that can be made in large batches for easy access during the busy week.

1. Low FODMAP Chicken & Vegetable Soup

Preparation time: 15 minutes
Cooking time: 45 minutes
Servings: 8

Ingredients:

- ☐ Two tbsp olive oil
- ☐ Two cups diced each carrots & celery
- ☐ One cup diced each green bell pepper & zucchini
- ☐ Eight cups chicken broth, low-sodium
- ☐ Four cups cooked chicken, shredded (preferably free-range or organic)
- ☐ Salt & pepper, as required

Directions:

1. Warm up oil in your big pot on moderate temp. Add carrots, celery, green bell pepper, and zucchini, then cook within fiver mins till vegetables are softened.
2. Add chicken broth, then let it boil. Adjust to a simmer within thirty mins. Mix in shredded cooked chicken, salt plus pepper, then simmer within ten mins. Serve.

Nutritional Values (per serving): Calories 181; Carbs 9g; Fat 8g; Protein 15g; Fiber 2g

NOTES

_____

_____

_____

2. SIBO-Friendly Turkey & Eggplant Casserole

Preparation time: 20 minutes
Cooking time: 45 minutes
Servings: 8

Ingredients:

- ☐ Two tbsp olive oil, divided
- ☐ One big eggplant, peeled & sliced into quarter-inch slices
- ☐ Salt & pepper, as required
- ☐ One-pound ground turkey (preferably free-range or organic)
- ☐ One cup diced each red bell pepper, zucchini & cherry tomatoes
- ☐ Two cups tomato sauce (low FODMAP, if needed)

Directions:

1. Warm up your oven to 375°F. Grease your big casserole dish with 1 tbsp oil.
2. Put eggplant slices on your baking sheet, then flavor it using salt plus pepper. Bake within 15 mins until slightly softened.
3. Meanwhile, in your big skillet on moderate-high temp, cook ground turkey in remaining oil. Add red bell pepper, zucchini, and cherry tomatoes, then cook till all vegetables are slightly softened.
4. In your prepared casserole dish, layer half of eggplant slices followed by half of turkey mixture. Top with half of the tomato sauce. Repeat layers once more.
5. Bake uncovered within 25 mins till bubbling around edges. Cool it down, then serve.

Nutritional Values (per serving): *Calories 239; Carbs 11g; Fat 14g; Protein 20g; Fiber 3g*

NOTES

_____

_____

_____

3. Turkey Meatballs with Zucchini Spaghetti

Preparation time: 15 minutes
Cooking time: 30 minutes
Servings: 4

Ingredients:

- ☐ One-pound ground turkey
- ☐ Half cup almond flour
- ☐ Quarter cup chopped parsley
- ☐ Quarter cup chopped green onion
- ☐ Salt & pepper, as required
- ☐ Two tbsp olive oil
- ☐ Four zucchini, spiralized into noodles & steamed

Directions:

1. In your container, mix ground turkey, almond flour, parsley, green onions, salt, and pepper. Form into meatballs.
2. Warm up oil in your big skillet on moderate temp. Add meatballs, then cook within 15 mins till browned. Serve zucchini noodles topped with cooked meatballs.

Nutritional Values (per serving): *Calories 425; Carbs 12g; Fat 23g; Protein 35g; Fiber 4g*

NOTES

_____

_____

_____

4. Creamy Coconut Cauliflower Soup

Preparation time: 10 minutes
Cooking time: 25 minutes
Servings: 6

Ingredients:

- One tbsp olive oil
- Half cup diced green onion
- One head cauliflower, chopped
- Four cups vegetable or chicken broth (low FODMAP)
- One cup canned coconut milk (full-fat)
- Salt & pepper, as required

Directions:

1. In your big pot, warm up oil on moderate temp. Put green onions, then cook till softened.
2. Add chopped cauliflower, then cook within 5 mins, mixing often. Pour in the broth, then let it boil. Simmer within 15 mins till cauliflower is tender.
3. Puree soup using your immersion blender till smooth. Mix in coconut milk, salt, plus pepper. Serve.

Nutritional Values (per serving): *Calories 150; Carbs 8g; Fat 12g; Protein 4g; Fiber 3g*

NOTES

_____

_____

_____

5. Slow-Cooker Chicken "Rice" Casserole

Preparation time: 10 minutes
Cooking time: 4 hours
Servings: 6

Ingredients:

- ☐ Two pounds no bones & skin chicken breasts, cubed
- ☐ Salt & pepper, as required
- ☐ Four cups riced cauliflower
- ☐ Half cup diced green onions
- ☐ Two cups low FODMAP tomato sauce
- ☐ Two tsp dried basil
- ☐ One tbsp olive oil

Directions:

1. Flavor cubed chicken using salt and pepper.
2. In your slow cooker, mix riced cauliflower, green onions, tomato sauce, and basil. Nestle the seasoned chicken cubes on top.
3. Drizzle with olive oil, then cover. Cook on LOW within four hours till chicken is cooked through. Serve.

Nutritional Values (per serving): Calories 300; Carbs 10g; Fat 8g; Protein 40g; Fiber 3g

NOTES

_____

_____

_____

These five recipes provide great options for batch cooking and freezing meals that are suitable for those dealing with SIBO. By taking the time to prepare these recipes ahead of time, you can ensure that you always have a nutritious and SIBO-friendly meal on hand.

Balancing Nutrition and Flavors In SIBO-Friendly Meals

Eating a diet tailored to managing Small Intestinal Bacterial Overgrowth (SIBO) can often feel restrictive, but it doesn't have to be boring or bland. Balancing nutrition and flavors in SIBO-friendly meals is possible with the right ingredients and techniques. With a bit of creativity, your dishes will not only be enjoyable but also compliant.

Though SIBO diets limit certain food groups, it's crucial to maintain a balanced intake of essential nutrients. Here are some tips for incorporating diverse nutrition while adhering to your dietary needs:

1. Consume protein-rich foods: Lean protein sources like chicken, turkey, or fish are recommended for those with SIBO. Well-cooked eggs (avoiding runny yolks) and tofu (for vegetarians/vegans) are also excellent protein options.

2. Incorporate low-FODMAP vegetables: A wide variety of vegetables is allowed on low-FODMAP diets. Focus on non-starchy options like leafy greens, zucchini, bell peppers, carrots, green beans, and cucumbers.

3. Prioritize healthy fats: Olive oil, avocado oil, and coconut oil are SIBO-friendly fats. Incorporate nuts and seeds like almonds, chia seeds, and pumpkin seeds in moderation.

4. Utilize alternative grains: Instead of wheat-based products, opt for healthier low-FODMAP grains such as quinoa, rice, and oats.

With the right seasonings and cooking techniques, you can create delicious and flavorful dishes that satisfy your taste buds without aggravating SIBO. Here are some ways to enhance flavors while staying compliant with your diet:

1. Experiment with herbs and spices: Fresh herbs like basil, cilantro, mint, parsley, rosemary, or thyme can significantly enhance the taste of SIBO-friendly dishes. Additionally, low-FODMAP spices like cumin, paprika, oregano, turmeric, and ginger can elevate the flavor profile.

2. Use citrus for a zesty punch: Lemons and limes are not only low-FODMAP but can also bring life to simple dishes by adding tanginess. Squeeze some fresh lemon or lime juice over salads, grilled fish or chicken dishes for a burst of freshness.

3. Roast or grill vegetables: Roasting or grilling vegetables caramelizes them and develops a depth of flavor that's hard to beat. Toss chopped veggies in olive oil and season with salt, pepper, and your favorite low-FODMAP herbs before roasting in the oven until tender.

4. Marinate proteins: Marinating meat or tofu can significantly improve taste while tenderizing the protein. Create a simple marinade using olive oil, lemon juice, Dijon mustard, garlic-infused oil (not minced garlic), salt, pepper, and your choice of herbs.

5. Make your sauces and dressings: Most store-bought condiments are high in FODMAPs; prepare homemade versions using low-FODMAP ingredients instead. Whip up a flavorful salad dressing by combining olive oil, lemon juice, salt, pepper, and your choice of herbs.

When it comes to balancing nutrition and flavors in SIBO-friendly meals, the key is experimenting with allowed ingredients to create satisfying and diverse dishes. While tackling SIBO with dietary changes might seem challenging at first, becoming more familiar with suitable foods will eventually lead you to create nutritious, delicious meals that keep both your taste buds and gut happy.

CHAPTER 7:
DINING OUT AND TRAVELING
ON THE SIBO DIET

Living with SIBO can be an uphill battle, but it doesn't have to take the fun out of eating out or attending social gatherings. By following a few tips and strategies, you can confidently navigate restaurants and social events with dietary restrictions while staying true to your SIBO diet.

1. Preparation is Key: Before heading out to a restaurant or social gathering, spend some time researching the establishment's menu online. Many restaurants offer detailed information about their dishes, and some even provide a separate menu for those with dietary restrictions. Familiarize yourself with the ingredients and make a mental note of any potential red flags.

2. Communicate your Needs: Don't be afraid to have an open conversation with the restaurant staff about your dietary restrictions. It's essential to let them know that you are on a SIBO diet and need to avoid specific foods. While not all servers may be familiar with SIBO, it's helpful if you provide them with a brief overview of your requirements.

3. Be Specific with your Order: When placing your order, be as detailed as possible about what you can and cannot eat. For instance, request gluten-free or low FODMAP menu items, ask the chef to avoid adding garlic or onion in your dish, and inquire about substitutions like using olive oil instead of butter.

4. Bring Digestive Enzymes: If you're worried that cross-contamination might occur in the kitchen, consider bringing digestive enzymes along with you. These enzymes can help you digest certain problematic foods more effectively and reduce the risk of experiencing discomfort during or after the meal.

5. Avoid Buffets: Buffets might seem like paradise to some, but they can be a nightmare for individuals on a strict diet plan like the SIBO diet. Cross-contamination is quite common at buffets, and it's challenging to know the exact ingredients of each dish. Stick to restaurants where you can order off a menu or attend gatherings with a catered meal.

6. Carry Snacks: Keeping a stash of SIBO-friendly snacks in your bag is always a good idea. These can include low FODMAP fruits, nuts, and seeds that provide a safe and nutritious alternative when there are no suitable options available at gatherings and restaurants.

7. Be the Host: Hosting dinner parties, potlucks, or social events at your home gives you full control over what's being served. You can either cook all the food yourself, adhering to your diet restrictions or ask guests to bring their favorite SIBO-friendly dishes along.

8. Make Smart Drink Choices: When it comes to beverages, choose wisely. Opt for water with lemon or lime, herbal teas, or low FODMAP smoothies instead of carbonated drinks or alcohol that might exacerbate your symptoms.

9. Find Support: Connect with others who have similar dietary restrictions through local support groups or online forums. Sharing experiences and exchanging tips on managing social situations while following a SIBO diet can prove invaluable.

10. Embrace the Positives: Remember that making good choices for your health is something to be proud of, even if it means skipping that delicious-looking dessert. Focus on enjoying the company of friends and family and savoring the SIBO-friendly foods available to you.

By planning ahead, communicating effectively with restaurant staff, making thoughtful choices when ordering and eating, carrying snacks along with digestive enzymes as needed, avoiding cross-contamination risks like buffets, hosting events that cater to your dietary needs, connecting with supportive communities, and remaining positive about your efforts – you can confidently enjoy dining out and attending social occasions while adhering to your SIBO diet.

Travel-Friendly SIBO Meals
And
Snacks

It is essential to plan and pack nutrition-packed meals and snacks while traveling, especially for individuals suffering from SIBO. Here are some travel-friendly SIBO meal and snack recipes to keep you satisfied and feeling well on your journey.

6. Coconut & Chia Overnight Oats

Preparation time: 5 minutes + chilling time
Cooking time: 0 minutes
Servings: 2

Ingredients:

- One cup rolled oats
- Two cups unsweetened coconut milk
- One tbsp chia seeds
- Half tsp vanilla extract
- Half cup of your favorite low-FODMAP berries (e.g. blueberries, strawberries)
- Two tbsp sliced almonds

Directions:

1. In your medium container, mix oats, coconut milk, chia seeds, plus vanilla extract.
2. Divide it into two separate glass jars, then top each serving with berries and sliced almonds. Refrigerate overnight, then take on travel.

Nutritional Values (per serving): *Calories 317; Carbs 39g; Fat 14g; Protein 10g; Fiber 8g*

NOTES

_____

_____

_____

7.Zucchini & Goat Cheese Frittata

Preparation time: 10 minutes
Cooking time: 15 minutes
Servings: 4

Ingredients:

- ☐ Six big eggs
- ☐ Three tbsp water
- ☐ Salt & black pepper, as required
- ☐ One tbsp olive oil
- ☐ Two medium zucchini, thinly sliced)
- ☐ Two oz crumbled goat cheese
- ☐ Two tbsp chopped fresh basil

Directions:

1. Warm up your oven to broil. In your big container, beat eggs with water, salt, plus pepper.
2. Warm up oil in your oven-safe pan on moderate temp. Add zucchini slices, then cook within five mins till tender.
3. Pour it on the cooked zucchini. Sprinkle with goat cheese plus basil. Cook on low temp within four mins till edges are set.
4. Transfer the pan to your oven, then broil within two to three mins till golden brown. Slice the frittata into four servings.

Nutritional Values (per serving): Calories 198; Carbs 4g; Fat 15g; Protein 13g; Fiber 1g

NOTES

_____

_____

_____

8. Quinoa Salad with Roasted Vegetables

Preparation time: 20 minutes
Cooking time: 25 minutes
Servings: 4

Ingredients:

- [ ] One cup uncooked quinoa, washed & strained
- [ ] Two cups water
- [ ] One tsp salt
- [ ] Two cups assorted bite-sized vegetables (zucchini, bell peppers, cherry tomatoes)
- [ ] Two tbsp olive oil
- [ ] Salt & pepper, as required
- [ ] Two tbsp fresh lemon juice

Directions:

1. Put quinoa in your medium saucepan with water plus salt. Let it boil, then adjust to low temp. Cover, then cook within 15 mins till tender. Remove, fluff it, then cool it down.
2. Warm up your oven to 425°F. Toss vegetables with oil, salt, plus pepper.
3. Spread them on your lined baking sheet. Roast within 25 mins till tender. Cool slightly before mixing them into quinoa. Add lemon juice, toss gently, then serve.

Nutritional Values (per serving): *Calories: 279; Carbs: 37g; Fat: 10g; Protein: 8g; Fiber: 6g*

NOTES

_____

_____

_____

9. Lemon Herb Chicken Salad Lettuce Wraps

Preparation time: 15 minutes
Cooking time: 0 minutes
Servings: 4

Ingredients:

- ☐ Two cups cooked shredded chicken
- ☐ One-third cup homemade or SIBO-friendly mayonnaise
- ☐ Juice & zest of one small lemon
- ☐ One tsp dried parsley flakes
- ☐ Salt & pepper, as required
- ☐ Eight large lettuce leaves (like romaine or butter lettuce)

Directions:

1. In your medium container, mix shredded chicken, mayonnaise, lemon juice, zest, parsley flakes, salt, plus pepper.
2. Put some chicken salad onto each lettuce leaf. Roll up the lettuce wraps and secure using toothpicks if desired. Serve.

__Nutritional Values (per serving):__ Calories: 207; Carbs: 2g; Fat: 12g; Protein: 22g; Fiber: 1g

NOTES

_____

_____

_____

10. Zucchini Noodle Pesto Pasta

Preparation time: 10 minutes
Cooking time: 0 minutes
Servings: 2

Ingredients:

- ☐ Two large zucchinis, spiralized
- ☐ One cup halved cherry tomatoes
- ☐ Half cup halved black olives
- ☐ Quarter cup pine nuts
- ☐ Half cup prepared pesto sauce (SIBO-friendly)

Directions:

1. Put spiralized zucchinis into your big container. Add cherry tomatoes, black olives, and pine nuts.
2. Add SIBO-friendly pesto sauce, then toss thoroughly. Serve.

Nutritional Values (per serving): *Calories: 420; Carbs: 16g; Fat: 36g; Protein: 9g; Fiber: 5g*

NOTES

_____

_____

_____

11. Veggie Wrap with Hummus and Avocado

Preparation time: 10 minutes
Cooking time: None
Servings: 2

Ingredients:

- ☐ Two big whole-grain tortillas or wraps
- ☐ Half cup hummus
- ☐ One small avocado, sliced
- ☐ One cup baby spinach leaves
- ☐ One medium thinly sliced red bell pepper
- ☐ One medium thinly sliced cucumber

Directions:

1. Lay out the tortillas on your clean surface, then spread each with half of hummus.
2. Layer avocado slices on top, then divide spinach leaves between both tortillas, then put them on top of avocado slices.
3. Add some bell pepper and cucumber slices to each tortilla. Carefully roll up each tortilla tightly, tucking in the sides as you go along.
4. Slice each wrap into halves or smaller sections if desired before serving.

Nutritional Values (per serving): *Calories: 335; Carbs: 45g; Fat: 13g; Protein: 11g; Fiber: 10g*

NOTES

_____

_____

_____

12. Spiced Chickpea Energy Bites

Preparation time: 15 minutes
Cooking time: 0 minutes
Servings: 12 bites

Ingredients:

- ☐ One & half cups cooked chickpeas, washed & strained
- ☐ Half cup almond butter
- ☐ Quarter cup maple syrup
- ☐ One tsp cinnamon
- ☐ Half tsp ginger powder
- ☐ Salt, as required

Directions:

1. Add chickpeas to your food processor, then blend till smooth.
2. Add almond butter, maple syrup, cinnamon, ginger powder, plus salt. Process again till smooth.
3. Scoop out portions of your dough, then roll into balls. Chill the energy bites in your fridge within 30 mins to set. Serve.

Nutritional Values (per serving): *Calories: 120; Carbs: 12g; Fat: 6g; Protein: 4g; Fiber: 2g*

NOTES

_____

_____

_____

13. SIBO-Friendly Trail Mix

Preparation time: 5 minutes
Cooking time: 0 minutes
Servings: 8

Ingredients:

- ☐ One cup unsalted almond
- ☐ One cup unsalted walnut
- ☐ One cup unsalted pumpkin seed
- ☐ Half cup unsweetened coconut flakes

Directions:

1. Mix all fixings in your big container.
2. Store the trail mix in your resealable bags for easy portioning and travel.

Nutritional Values (per serving): *Calories 389; Carbs 9g; Fat 36g; Protein 15g; Fiber 4g*

NOTES

_____

_____

_____

14. Almond Butter Stuffed Dates

Preparation time: 10 minutes
Cooking time: 0 minutes
Servings: 12 stuffed dates

Ingredients:

- ☐ Twelve pitted Medjool dates, sliced a small slit on one side
- ☐ Half cup almond butter, unsweetened
- ☐ Two ounces dark chocolate, melted

Directions:

1. Carefully fill each date with two tsp almond butter. Put stuffed dates on your lined tray lined.
2. Drizzle melted dark chocolate over each almond butter stuffed date. Refrigerate the dates within 20 minutes till chocolate has hardened. Serve.

Nutritional Values (per serving): *Calories: 175; Carbs: 25g; Fat: 7g; Protein: 2g; Fiber: 2g*

NOTES

_____

_____

_____

15. Almond Butter Energy Bites

Preparation time: 10 minutes

Chilling time: 20 minutes

Servings: 12

Ingredients:

- ☐ One cup rolled oats
- ☐ Half cup natural almond butter
- ☐ Quarter cup honey
- ☐ Half cup unsweetened coconut flakes
- ☐ Two tbsp chia seeds
- ☐ Half tsp vanilla extract

Directions:

1. In your big container, mix rolled oats, almond butter, honey, coconut flakes, chia seeds, and vanilla. Shape the mixture into small balls.
2. Put energy bites onto your parchment-lined baking sheet, then chill within 20 minutes in your refrigerator to firm up.

Nutritional Values (per serving): Calories: 140; Carbs: 13g; Fat: 8g; Protein: 4g; Fiber: 3g

NOTES

_____

_____

_____

Communicating Your Dietary Needs Effectively

If you're on the SIBO diet, it can be challenging to navigate dining out and travel while maintaining your dietary restrictions. However, communicating your needs effectively can ensure that you enjoy delicious meals without compromising your digestive health. Let's explore some tips for discussing your dietary needs with restaurant staff and making the best choices while dining out or traveling.

1. Be prepared: Before going to a restaurant or traveling to a new destination, research the venues in advance to find ones that can cater to your specific dietary needs. Look for menus online, read reviews from other diners with similar diets, or call the restaurant directly to inquire about their ability to accommodate your restrictions.

2. Be concise and clear: When communicating with restaurant staff or vendors, avoid complicated medical jargon or technical terms related to SIBO. Instead, focus on explaining your dietary needs in simple layman language. For instance, you may say something like, "I need a meal free of garlic, onions, and certain types of carbohydrates."

3. Use allergy cards: Create a small laminated card that outlines your dietary restrictions in bullet points. You can hand it to the waiter as you explain your needs verbally. It will make it easier for them to remember and communicate with kitchen staff as they prepare your food.

4. Practice cultural sensitivity when traveling: When traveling abroad, learning a few key phrases in the local language related to your dietary needs would be helpful. Research any cultural differences that may affect how locals understand and respond to your requests – this will ensure smooth communication and a better dining experience.

5. Prioritize communication over perfection.: While it's crucial to advocate for yourself and ensure adherence to your SIBO diet as much as possible, recognize that mistakes may happen due to miscommunications or restaurant staff unfamiliarity with your dietary needs. Instead of becoming upset, remain patient and continue educating those around you about your requirements.

6. Be open to alternatives: In some cases, the restaurant may not have a dish that meets your dietary needs. Consider asking the chef if they can make you something off-menu with ingredients that you know are safe for your diet.

7. Make use of technology: There are numerous smartphone apps that can translate your dietary needs into multiple languages, convert ingredient lists to SIBO-friendly recipes, and even point out local restaurants that cater to special diets. Utilize these tools to make dining out and traveling easier while on the SIBO diet.

8. Bring backup: If you're traveling, pack some SIBO-friendly snacks or a meal in case you cannot find options at your destination. This can relieve stress and ensure you have something safe to eat when necessary.

9. Show appreciation: When servers or chefs go above and beyond to accommodate your dietary needs, express gratitude through verbal appreciation or tips in countries where it's customary.

10. Share your experiences: Leaving reviews on online platforms like Yelp or TripAdvisor can help other SIBO-diagnosed individuals find restaurants that are sensitive to their requirements. Share both positive and negative experiences so others can benefit from your insight.

11. Plan social events carefully: If you're hosting friends or attending gatherings, communicate with the organizers beforehand so they can prepare food suitable for your diet – this will ensure you feel included while maintaining your health priorities.

12. Educate yourself on SIBO-friendly dishes: The more you know about what ingredients and dishes are usually safe for those on the SIBO diet, the better equipped you'll be to make informed decisions in various dining settings.

Remember that communication is key when it comes to maintaining a healthy lifestyle with SIBO restrictions while dining out or traveling. Patience, preparation, and persistence will help you navigate the challenges of adhering to your diet while still enjoying the social aspect of sharing meals with others.

CHAPTER 8:
COPING WITH EMOTIONAL EATING AND STRESS

Emotional eating is a behavior where people use food to cope with emotional triggers such as stress, anger, or sadness. It often involves consuming large quantities of unhealthy foods, which can lead to weight gain and other health issues. For people with SIBO, emotional eating can cause additional discomfort as it may increase digestive issues and perpetuate anxiety around symptoms.

SIBO symptoms contribute to intensified stress levels due to their impact on daily life routines and social interactions. Stress can also worsen SIBO by altering gut motility and impacting the immune system.

Hence, managing stress and reversing emotional eating habits are essential in dealing with SIBO effectively.

Addressing Emotional Triggers for Overeating

It is important for those with SIBO to follow a specific diet and treatment plan to alleviate their symptoms. However, overcoming emotional triggers that lead to overeating can be a significant challenge.

Overeating can exacerbate the symptoms of SIBO and derail one's progress toward improving gut health. This section aims to address the emotional triggers for overeating in SIBO patients and provide strategies for overcoming them.

1. Stress: Stress is one of the most common emotional triggers for overeating. When individuals feel overwhelmed by work, relationships, or other life challenges, they may turn to food for comfort. In many cases, this results in consuming large quantities of food that can further irritate the gut.

To better handle stress without overeating:

☐ Incorporate relaxation techniques such as deep breathing exercises, yoga, or meditation into your daily routine.

☐ Seek support from friends or family members when you feel overwhelmed.

☐ Break bigger tasks into smaller steps to make them more manageable.

☐ Maintain a healthy work-life balance.

2. Anxiety: Anxiety can prompt overeating as it often leads individuals to crave high-calorie, carbohydrate-rich foods which may exacerbate SIBO symptoms. Moreover, these anxiety-induced cravings may not necessarily be for healthy options.

Here are some ways to alleviate anxiety without overeating:

- ☐ Engage in regular physical activity to release endorphins and reduce anxiety.
- ☐ Avoid caffeine and excessive sugar consumption that may worsen anxiety.
- ☐ Practice mindfulness techniques such as deep breathing and visualization to manage anxiety levels.
- ☐ Consult with a mental health professional if you require additional support.

3. Boredom: Boredom can easily lead to overeating as individuals search for ways to pass the time, satisfy cravings, or seek a sense of enjoyment from food. Overeating during boredom may not involve symptoms of hunger, but rather a desire for pleasurable sensations or distractions.

To address the impact of boredom on overeating:

- ☐ Develop and engage in hobbies or activities you enjoy.
- ☐ Create and maintain a daily routine to prevent excessive downtime.
- ☐ Refrain from consuming SIBO-triggering foods while watching television or engaging in other mindless activities.
- ☐ Socialize with friends and family members through phone calls or video chats to stay connected and reduce boredom-driven eating.

4. Emotional Eating: Healthy individuals may experience emotional eating occasionally, but for those with SIBO, excessive emotional eating can worsen their condition. People may eat more when they are sad, lonely, angry, or even happy.

To overcome emotional eating habits:

- ☐ Keep a food diary to track your emotions and the types of food you eat in response to these emotions.
- ☐ Recognize your emotional triggers and develop alternative coping strategies such as exercising, reading, or listening to music.
- ☐ Practice mindfulness-based techniques like meditation and deep breathing to improve emotional stability.
- ☐ Seek support from friends, family members, or a therapist to discuss your emotional triggers.

5. Eating Out of Habit: SIBO sufferers may eat out of habit, engaging in mindless snacking at specific times of the day or during certain activities. To break this cycle:

- ☐ Establish new habits around food consumption by setting specific meal times and sticking with them.
- ☐ Remove trigger foods from your environment that may entice habitual overeating.

☐ Replace unhealthy snacking habits with healthier ones centered around permitted SIBO-friendly foods.

☐ Slow down when eating and listen to your body's hunger cues instead of eating out of habit.

Addressing emotional triggers for overeating is a vital component of managing SIBO effectively. By recognizing and targeting the root causes of emotional eating, individuals can take charge of their habits and improve their overall gut health.

Mindful Eating Practices for SIBO Management

One crucial aspect of managing SIBO is adopting mindful eating practices. Being mindful when eating is an essential part of your overall healing journey while living with SIBO. It can help you recognize your body's hunger and fullness cues, improve digestion, reduce stress, and make healthier meal choices. Here are some practical mindful eating practices to aid in SIBO management:

1. Eat Slowly: Taking the time to eat slowly allows you to savor each bite and chew thoroughly. This not only helps to break down food more effectively but also gives your body time to send signals of satiety to your brain before overeating occurs. Try setting a timer for 20-30 minutes for each meal and focus on taking smaller bites.

2. Limit Distractions: To practice mindful eating, eliminate distractions such as television screens, phones, or computers during meals. These distractions can pull your attention away from your food and contribute to mindless or emotional eating patterns that trigger SIBO symptoms. Instead, focus solely on your meal and engage all your senses while eating.

3. Listen to Your Body: Becoming more aware of hunger signals and learning the difference between physical hunger and emotional cravings are valuable skills in SIBO management. Before reaching for food, take a moment to assess whether you're truly hungry or simply feeling bored or stressed. By learning to listen to your body's needs better, you'll be able to make wiser decisions about what, when, and how much you eat.

4. Keep a Food Diary: Recording your meals and observing the way they affect your body helps you become more aware of which foods and eating patterns exacerbate your SIBO symptoms. A food diary can be a valuable source of information to help you and your healthcare provider determine appropriate dietary modifications.

5. Practice Gratitude: Before eating, take a moment to express gratitude for the food on your plate. Giving thanks can help create a positive mindset around mealtime and shift your focus to nourishing your body with healthful choices.

6. Make Mindful Food Choices: Choose foods that promote gut health and minimize SIBO symptoms when planning your meals. Foods rich in fiber, such as fruits, vegetables, and whole grains, are beneficial to gut health. Consult with your healthcare provider for specific dietary recommendations tailored to your unique needs.

7. Balance Your Plate: Aim for a balance between macronutrients (protein, carbohydrates, and fats) and micronutrients (vitamins and minerals) on your plate. This balance promotes optimal digestion while providing the necessary nourishment for healing from SIBO.

8. Practice Portion Control: Overeating contributes to gastrointestinal distress and exacerbates SIBO symptoms. To minimize this risk, make a conscious effort to control portion sizes by using smaller plates or measuring cups to serve food.

9. Prioritize Hydration: Drinking enough water is essential for promoting proper digestion and overall well-being while managing SIBO. Aim for at least 8-10 glasses of water per day to support optimal hydration levels.

10. Address Emotional Eating: Stress, anxiety, or other negative emotions often lead to emotional eating fueled by comfort rather than actual hunger. Developing healthy coping mechanisms, such as journaling, deep breathing exercises, or seeking professional support can help address emotional eating behaviors.

Incorporating mindful eating practices into your daily routine will not only improve digestion but also create a more harmonious relationship with food. By becoming more present and aware during mealtimes, you can be empowered to make dietary choices that support your SIBO management journey, ultimately leading to better health and well-being.

Stress-Reduction Techniques for Better Gut Health

While some stress is unavoidable, constant exposure to it can adversely impact our health, especially gut health. Studies have demonstrated that stress plays a significant role in the development and aggravation of gut-related issues, including Small Intestinal Bacterial Overgrowth (SIBO). There are several stress-reduction techniques you can adopt to foster better gut health in SIBO management. These methods may not only alleviate your symptoms but also enhance your quality of life.

1. Mindfulness Meditation: Studies have shown that mindfulness meditation is an effective way to combat stress and promote relaxation. This practice involves focusing on breath control and mental awareness to cultivate a state of mindfulness in daily life. Practicing mindfulness meditation regularly can help regulate the balance between your sympathetic and parasympathetic nervous systems, thereby improving gut functioning.

2. Yoga: Yoga combines physical postures with breathing exercises and meditation to enhance relaxation and reduce anxiety. These stretches and movements stimulate the digestive system by promoting blood flow to your organs while also relieving muscular tension in your abdomen. Incorporating yoga into your routine may prove beneficial for reducing stress related to SIBO.

3. Exercise: Engaging in regular physical activity not only improves cardiovascular health but also releases endorphins, the so-called "feel-good" hormones. These hormones combat stress and promote a sense of well-being. Research suggests that regular exercise can help improve gut health through better circulation and digestion.

4. Sleep: Prioritizing sleep is another way to manage stress and maintain a healthy gut. Disrupted sleep patterns can negatively impact the balance of your nervous system, exacerbating SIBO symptoms. Create an optimal sleep environment by sticking to a consistent bedtime, reducing blue light exposure before bed, and establishing a calming bedtime routine.

5. Deep Breathing Exercises: Deep breathing exercises are effective in managing stress because they help stimulate the parasympathetic nervous system, which promotes relaxation and enhances digestion. Try activities like diaphragmatic breathing, box breathing, or alternate nostril breathing to help lower stress levels.

6. Counseling or Psychotherapy: In cases where stress becomes overwhelming or unmanageable, it might be beneficial to seek professional help from a counselor or therapist trained in stress management techniques. Cognitive-behavioral therapy (CBT) is an example of a therapeutic approach that has been proven effective in addressing stress-related issues.

7. Social Support: Building and maintaining strong connections with friends and family members can provide essential emotional support during times of stress. Research shows that individuals with strong social networks tend to have lower stress levels and improved gut health.

8. Nutrition: Ensuring a nutrient-rich diet can also aid in combating stress by providing essential vitamins and minerals required for proper bodily functioning. Consider incorporating probiotics, prebiotics, and fermented foods that promote a healthy gut microbiome.

9. Relaxation Techniques: Engaging in various relaxation techniques such as progressive muscle relaxation, visualization, and self-hypnosis can help reduce stress and promote a sense of calm. Implement these practices daily or as needed to manage stress levels effectively.

10. Time Management: Assessing and managing your time wisely can prevent overwhelming situations that contribute to stress. Prioritize tasks, break them into smaller achievable goals, and delegate when necessary to maintain a balanced, stress-free life.

Adopting one or more stress-reduction techniques can significantly impact SIBO management by promoting better gut health. Adopting a comprehensive approach that addresses both mental and physical well-being is crucial for successfully managing SIBO symptoms and leading a healthier life.

CHAPTER 9:
SIBO-FRIENDLY
FAMILY MEALS

16. Baked Salmon with Lemon and Dill

Preparation time: 15 minutes
Cooking time: 20 minutes
Servings: 4

Ingredients:

- ☐ Four (six-oz) salmon fillets, pat dried
- ☐ One tbsp olive oil
- ☐ One tsp sea salt
- ☐ Half tsp black pepper, ground
- ☐ One lemon, thinly sliced
- ☐ Six sprigs of fresh dill

Directions:

1. Warm up your oven to 425°F.
2. Put salmon fillets on your lined baking sheet. Drizzle each fillet using oil, then flavor with sea salt plus black pepper.
3. Put two to three lemon slices on top. Arrange a fresh dill sprig on lemon slices. Bake within 15 to 20 mins till salmon is cooked through. Serve.

Nutritional Values (per serving): *Calories: 300; Carbs: 2g; Fat: 19g; Protein: 24g; Fiber: 1g*

NOTES

_____

_____

_____

17. Grilled Chicken with Herbs and Zucchini Noodles

Preparation time: 15 minutes
Cooking time: 14 minutes
Servings: 4

Ingredients:

- [ ] Four no bones & skin chicken breasts
- [ ] One tbsp garlic-infused olive oil
- [ ] Two tbsp chopped basil, fresh
- [ ] Two tbsp chopped parsley, fresh
- [ ] One tsp dried each oregano & rosemary
- [ ] One tsp salt
- [ ] Half tsp black pepper
- [ ] Four medium zucchinis, spiralized into noodles
- [ ] One tbsp olive oil

Directions:

1. Warm up your grill to moderate-high temp.
2. In your small container, mix garlic-infused olive oil, basil, parsley, oregano, rosemary, salt, and pepper. Rub it onto each chicken breast till coated.
3. Put chicken breasts on your grill, then cook within seven mins per side till fully cooked through. Remove, then cool it down before slicing.
4. Warm up one oil in your big skillet on moderate temp. Add spiralized zucchini noodles, then cook within 3-4 mins, mixing often.
5. Divide zucchini noodles among four plates. Top each plate with a sliced grilled chicken breast.

Nutritional Values (per serving): *Calories: 297; Carbs: 10g; Fat: 14g; Protein: 34g; Fiber: 3g*

NOTES

_____

_____

18. Garlic Shrimp and Broccoli Stir-Fry

Preparation time: 15 minutes
Cooking time: 10 minutes
Servings: 4

Ingredients:

- [ ] One-pound medium shrimp, peeled & cleaned
- [ ] Two cups broccoli florets
- [ ] Three tbsp garlic-infused olive oil, divided
- [ ] One tbsp lemon juice
- [ ] One tbsp soy sauce, low-sodium (gluten-free if needed)
- [ ] Half tsp black pepper, ground
- [ ] Half tsp salt
- [ ] Two tsp cornstarch
- [ ] Half cup water

Directions:

1. In your small container, whisk lemon juice, soy sauce, salt, plus black pepper. Put aside. In your separate container, mix cornstarch and water. Put aside.
2. Heat two tbsp garlic-infused olive oil in your big skillet on moderate-high temp.
3. Add shrimp, then cook within 2 to 3 mins on each side till they turn pink. Remove, then put aside.
4. In your same skillet, add remaining garlic-infused olive oil on moderate-high temp. Add broccoli florets, then cook for 5 to 6 minutes till tender.
5. Add cooked shrimp, then pour in lemon juice mixture. Mix well. Mix in cornstarch mixture slowly while mixing within 1-2 mins till sauce has thickened. Serve.

Nutritional Values (per serving): *Calories: 230; Carbs: 12g; Fat: 10g; Protein: 24g; Fiber: 2g*

NOTES

_____

_____

19. Lemon-Herb Roasted Turkey Breast

Preparation time: 20 minutes
Cooking time: 1 hour & 30 minutes
Servings: 6

Ingredients:

- [ ] One & half pounds no bones & skin turkey breast, pat dried
- [ ] One big lemon, zested & juiced
- [ ] Three tbsp olive oil
- [ ] Two tbsp thyme, chopped
- [ ] Two tbsp rosemary, chopped
- [ ] One tbsp ground black pepper
- [ ] Half tbsp salt

Directions:

1. Warm up your oven to 350°F.
2. In your small container, mix zest, juice, oil, thyme, rosemary, black pepper, plus salt.
3. Put turkey breast on your foil-lined baking sheet. Pour lemon-herb mixture on top.
4. Roast within 1 hour and 30 mins, basting with juices every 30 mins. Remove, cool it down, slice, then serve.

Nutritional Values (per serving): Calories: 290; Carbs: 2g; Fat: 12g; Protein: 40g; Fiber: 1g

NOTES

_____

_____

_____

20. Spaghetti Squash with Tomato Basil Sauce

Preparation time: 15 minutes
Cooking time: 45 minutes
Servings: 4

Ingredients:

- ☐ One medium-sized spaghetti squash, halved lengthwise & seeded
- ☐ Two cups canned crushed tomatoes (no onion or garlic)
- ☐ One tbsp olive oil
- ☐ Half cup chopped fresh basil leaves
- ☐ Salt & pepper, as required
- ☐ One tbsp garlic-infused oil (for low-FODMAP)

Directions:

1. Warm up your oven to 375°F. Put squash on your lined baking sheet.
2. Bake within 40-45 mins till squash is tender. Cool it down, then shred it into spaghetti-like strands.
3. In your medium saucepan, warm up oil on low temp. Add garlic-infused oil, then warm it up. Add crushed tomatoes, mixing often till heated through.
4. Add basil leaves, salt, plus pepper, then simmer within 10 minutes. Divide spaghetti squash among four plates, then spoon tomato basil sauce on top. Serve.

Nutritional Values (per serving): Calories: 130; Carbs: 19g; Fat: 6g; Protein: 4g; Fiber: 4g

NOTES

_____

_____

_____

21. Turkey and Vegetable Meatballs

Preparation time: 20 minutes
Cooking time: 30 minutes
Servings: 4

Ingredients:

- [ ] One pound ground turkey
- [ ] One half cup grated carrot
- [ ] One half cup grated zucchini
- [ ] Two tbsp chopped each chives & parsley
- [ ] One tbsp garlic-infused olive oil (strictly from the infused oil no solids)
- [ ] One large egg, beaten
- [ ] Three fourths cup almond flour
- [ ] One tsp dried oregano
- [ ] Salt & pepper, as required

Directions:

1. Warm up your oven to 400°F.
2. In your big container, mix ground turkey, grated carrot, grated zucchini, chopped chives, chopped parsley, garlic-infused olive oil, plus beaten egg.
3. Add almond flour, dried oregano, salt, plus pepper. Mix well. Shape it into even-sized meatballs, the put them on your lined baking sheet.
4. Bake within 25 to 30 mins till lightly browned. Remove, cool it down, then serve.

Nutritional Values (per serving): *Calories: 350; Carbs: 12g; Fat: 24g; Protein: 25g; Fiber: 3g*

NOTES

_____

_____

_____

22. Pan-Seared Cod with Cilantro Lime Sauce

Preparation time: 15 minutes
Cooking time: 10 minutes
Servings: 4

Ingredients:

- [ ] Four (six-oz) Cod fillets, washed & pat dried
- [ ] One tsp kosher salt
- [ ] Half tsp black pepper
- [ ] One tbsp garlic-infused olive oil
- [ ] One tbsp unsalted butter
- [ ] One-fourth cup chopped cilantro
- [ ] Zest of one lime
- [ ] Two tbsp lime juice
- [ ] One-fourth cup chopped scallions (green parts only)
- [ ] Three tbsp mayonnaise
- [ ] One tsp Dijon mustard

Directions:

1. Flavor the cod fillets using kosher salt plus black pepper. Warm up garlic-infused olive oil plus butter in your big skillet on moderate-high temp.
2. Put seasoned cod fillets in your skillet, then cook within 4-5 mins on each side till fish is cooked through.
3. Meanwhile, whisk cilantro, zest, juice, scallions, mayonnaise, and Dijon mustard in your medium container. Drizzle each fillet with cilantro-lime sauce. Serve.

Nutritional Values (per serving): *Calories: 285; Carbs: 2g; Fat: 17g; Protein: 31g; Fiber: 0.7g*

NOTES

_____

_____

23. Lemon Garlic Roasted Asparagus

Preparation time: 10 minutes
Cooking time: 15 minutes
Servings: 4

Ingredients:

- [ ] 16 trimmed asparagus spears
- [ ] One tbsp garlic-infused olive oil
- [ ] Half tsp ground black pepper
- [ ] Half tsp sea salt
- [ ] Zest of two lemons
- [ ] Two tbsp lemon juice

Directions:

1. Warm up your oven to 400°F.
2. In your small container, whisk garlic-infused olive oil, zest, juice, salt, plus pepper. Put asparagus spears on your baking sheet, then drizzle with lemon garlic mixture. Toss well.
3. Roast within 12-15 mins till tender. Serve.

Nutritional Values (per serving): *Calories: 60; Carbs: 4g; Fat: 5g; Protein: 2g; Fiber: 1g*

NOTES

_____

_____

_____

24. Balsamic Glazed Chicken Thighs

Preparation time: 15 minutes
Cooking time: 45 minutes
Servings: 4

Ingredients:

- [ ] Eight bone-in, skin-on chicken thighs
- [ ] One-fourth cup garlic-infused olive oil
- [ ] Three-fourths cup balsamic vinegar
- [ ] Two tbsp pure maple syrup
- [ ] Two tbsp Dijon mustard (SIBO-friendly)
- [ ] One tbsp chopped fresh thyme
- [ ] Half tsp Himalayan salt
- [ ] One-fourth tsp black pepper

Directions:

1. Warm up your oven to 400°F. In your small container, mix garlic-infused olive oil, vinegar, maple syrup, mustard, thyme, salt, plus pepper.
2. Put chicken thighs on your parchment-lined baking sheet. Pour balsamic mixture on chicken thighs till coated.
3. Bake within 25 mins, remove, then baste each thigh with more balsamic glaze. Bake again within 20 mins till fully cooked through. Serve.

Nutritional Values (per serving): *Calories: 450; Carbs: 12g; Fat: 34g; Protein: 25g; Fiber: 0g*

NOTES

_____

_____

_____

25. Sautéed Spinach with Garlic and Pine Nuts

Preparation time: 10 minutes
Cooking time: 5 minutes
Servings: 4

Ingredients:

- ☐ Four cups fresh spinach, washed & strained
- ☐ Two tbsp garlic-infused olive oil
- ☐ One-third cup pine nuts
- ☐ Half tsp sea salt
- ☐ Quarter tsp black pepper, ground
- ☐ Two tsp lemon juice

Directions:

1. Warm up garlic-infused olive oil in your big skillet on moderate temp. Add pine nuts, then cook them within two mins till lightly golden brown.
2. Add spinach, then cook it within 2-3 minutes till it wilts. Flavor spinach using sea salt plus black pepper. Remove your skillet, then drizzle lemon juice on the spinach. Serve.

Nutritional Values (per serving): *Calories: 138; Carbs: 3g; Fat: 13g; Protein: 2g; Fiber: 1g*

NOTES

_____

_____

_____

26. Roasted Cauliflower and Brussels Sprouts

Preparation time: 15 minutes
Cooking time: 25 minutes
Servings: 4

Ingredients:

- ☐ One small head cauliflower, c florets
- ☐ Two cups trimmed & halved Brussels sprouts
- ☐ Three tbsp olive oil
- ☐ One tsp garlic-infused oil
- ☐ One tsp dried thyme
- ☐ One tsp dried rosemary
- ☐ Half tsp ground black pepper
- ☐ Half tsp sea salt

Directions:

1. Warm up your oven to 425°F. In your big container, add cauliflower florets and Brussels sprouts.
2. In your small container, whisk olive oil, garlic-infused oil, thyme, rosemary, black pepper, plus sea salt. Pour oil mixture on the vegetables, then toss well.
3. Spread vegetables on your lined baking sheet. Roast within 25 minutes, flipping once, till vegetables are tender. Remove, cool it down, then serve.

Nutritional Values (per serving): *Calories: 145; Carbs: 12g; Fat: 10g; Protein: 4g; Fiber: 5g*

NOTES

_____

_____

_____

27. Rosemary and Thyme Roasted Chicken

Preparation time: 20 minutes
Cooking time: 1 hour & 30 minutes
Servings: 4

Ingredients:

- ☐ One whole chicken (approximately four pounds), pat dried
- ☐ Two tbsp olive oil
- ☐ Two tsp rosemary, chopped, fresh
- ☐ Two tsp thyme, chopped, fresh
- ☐ One tsp garlic-infused olive oil
- ☐ One tsp sea salt
- ☐ Half tsp black pepper
- ☐ Two cups diced carrots
- ☐ Two cups diced zucchini

Directions:

1. Warm up your oven to 375°F.
2. In your small container, mix oil, rosemary, thyme, garlic-infused olive oil, salt, plus pepper.
3. Carefully loosen the skin above the breast meat to create pockets. Spread about two-thirds marinade under the chicken skin.
4. Rub remaining marinade on the entire outside surface of your chicken. Tuck both wings under the chicken.
5. Put whole marinated chicken on your roasting tray. Scatter diced carrots and zucchini around the chicken.
6. Roast within 1 hour and 30 minutes till cooked through, basting with pan juices often. Cool it down, carve, then serve.

Nutritional Values (per serving): *Calories: 572; Carbs: 10g; Fat: 30g; Protein: 54g; Fiber: 3g*

NOTES

_____

_____

28. Zucchini and Carrot Fritters

Preparation time: 15 minutes
Cooking time: 8 minutes
Servings: 4

Ingredients:

- ☐ One medium grated zucchini
- ☐ Two medium carrots, grated
- ☐ Third cup all-purpose flour, gluten-free
- ☐ Half tsp baking powder
- ☐ Quarter tsp salt
- ☐ Quarter tsp of pepper
- ☐ One large egg, lightly beaten
- ☐ Two tbsp garlic-infused oil (green parts only)

Directions:

1. In your big container, mix grated zucchini and carrots.
2. In your separate container, mix flour, baking powder, salt, plus pepper. Add it to zucchini and carrot mixture, then mix well. Mix in beaten egg till blended.
3. Warm up garlic-infused oil in your non-stick frying pan on moderate temp. Drop some fritter batter into your pan, then flatten slightly.
4. Cook within four mins per side till golden brown. Repeat steps with remaining batter. Serve.

Nutritional Values (per serving): *Calories: 210; Carbs: 24g; Fat: 10g; Protein: 5g; Fiber: 2g*

NOTES

_____

_____

_____

29. Grilled Steak with Chimichurri Sauce

Preparation time: 20 minutes
Cooking time: 10 minutes
Servings: 4

Ingredients:

- ☐ Four (six-oz) beef steaks (such as sirloin or ribeye), about an inch thick
- ☐ Two tbsp garlic-infused olive oil, divided
- ☐ One tsp ground black pepper
- ☐ One tsp sea salt
- ☐ One cup Italian flat-leaf parsley, chopped
- ☐ Half cup cilantro, chopped
- ☐ Two tbsp red wine vinegar
- ☐ Two tbsp lemon juice
- ☐ Half tsp ground cumin
- ☐ Quarter cup olive oil

Directions:

1. Warm up your grill to high temp.
2. Rub steaks with one tbsp garlic-infused olive oil, then flavor them with salt plus pepper.
3. In your container, mix remaining garlic-infused olive oil, parsley, cilantro, vinegar, juice, and cumin. Whisk in olive oil till chimichurri sauce. Put aside.
4. Grill steaks within 4 to 5 mins per side till cooked through. Remove, then cool it down. Slice steaks against the grain, then serve with chimichurri sauce on top.

Nutritional Values (per serving): *Calories: 565; Carbs: 3g; Fat: 43g; Protein: 42g; Fiber: 1g*

NOTES

_____

_____

_____

30. Stuffed Bell Peppers with Ground Turkey

Preparation time: 20 minutes
Cooking time: 45 minutes
Servings: 4

Ingredients:

- [ ] Four medium-sized bell peppers, any color, tops removed & seeds discarded
- [ ] One pound ground turkey
- [ ] Half cup cooked long-grain rice (white or brown)
- [ ] One large carrot, finely grated
- [ ] Two tbsp olive oil
- [ ] One tsp dried each basil & oregano
- [ ] Half tsp salt
- [ ] Quarter tsp ground black pepper
- [ ] Half cup grated low-FODMAP cheese (such as cheddar, Colby, or parmesan)
- [ ] Two cups low-FODMAP marinara sauce

Directions:

1. Warm up your oven to 350°F.
2. In your big container, mix ground turkey, cooked rice, grated carrot, dried basil, dried oregano, salt, plus black pepper. Divide turkey mixture among your four hollowed-out bell peppers.
3. In your small container, mix marinara sauce plus one tbsp olive oil. Pour a quarter of marinara sauce mixture on each stuffed bell pepper.
4. Put stuffed bell peppers in your baking dish, then drizzle with remaining olive oil. Bake within 35 to 40 mins till cooked through.
5. Remove, then sprinkle each pepper with grated cheese. Bake again within 5 mins till cheese is melted. Remove, cool it down, then serve.

Nutritional Values (per serving): *Calories: 450; Carbs: 30g; Fat: 25g; Protein: 30g; Fiber: 4g*

NOTES

_____

_____

31. Baked Eggplant Parmesan

Preparation time: 20 minutes
Cooking time: 35 minutes
Servings: 4

Ingredients:

- [ ] One big eggplant, sliced into 1/4-inch-thick rounds
- [ ] Three-quarters cup almond flour
- [ ] One-half cup grated parmesan cheese
- [ ] One tsp Italian seasoning
- [ ] One-half tsp salt
- [ ] One-fourth tsp black pepper
- [ ] Two large eggs
- [ ] Two cups low-FODMAP marinara sauce (e.g., FODY Foods brand)
- [ ] One cup shredded mozzarella cheese

Directions:

1. Warm up your oven to 400°F.
2. Put eggplant slices on paper towels, then sprinkle with salt. Let it sit within 10 mins to draw out moisture, wipe off excess salt, then pat them dry.
3. In your shallow container, mix almond flour, grated parmesan cheese, Italian seasoning, salt, plus black pepper. In another shallow container, beat the eggs.
4. Dip each eggplant slice into beaten eggs, then coat with almond flour mixture. Put breaded eggplant slices on your lined baking sheet.
5. Bake eggplant slices on your center rack within 15 minutes, flip them, then bake within 15 mins till crispy. Adjust your oven temperature to 375°F.
6. Spread some low-FODMAP marinara sauce in your eight-by-eight-inch baking dish. Layer half of baked eggplant slices, followed by another layer of marinara, and half of mozzarella.
7. Repeat with another layer of eggplant slices, sauce, and remaining mozzarella cheese. Bake within 20-25 mins till bubbly. Remove, cool it down, then serve.

Nutritional Values (per serving): *Calories: 329; Carbs: 19g; Fat: 19g; Protein: 23g; Fiber: 6g*

NOTES

_____

_____

32. Lemon-Herb Grilled Shrimp Skewers

Preparation time: 15 minutes
Cooking time: 10 minutes
Servings: 4

Ingredients:

- ☐ Two pounds big shrimp, peeled & cleaned
- ☐ Quarter cup garlic-infused olive oil
- ☐ One tbsp fresh lemon juice
- ☐ Two tsp lemon zest
- ☐ One tbsp chopped each thyme & parsley
- ☐ One tsp ground black pepper
- ☐ Half tsp salt

Directions:

1. In your small container, mix garlic-infused olive oil, juice, zest, thyme, parsley, black pepper, plus salt.
2. Put shrimp in your big resealable bag, then pour marinade. Marinate within 10 mins in your fridge.
3. Warm up your grill to moderate-high temp. Thread marinated shrimp onto your metal skewers.
4. Put shrimp skewers on your grill, then cook within 4-5 mins per side till they turn pink. Serve.

Nutritional Values (per serving): *Calories: 391; Carbs: 2g; Fat: 21g; Protein: 47g; Fiber: 0g*

NOTES

_____

_____

_____

33. Turkey and Vegetable Stir-Fry

Preparation time: 15 minutes
Cooking time: 15 minutes
Servings: 4

Ingredients:

- One-pound diced turkey breast
- One medium chopped each red bell pepper & zucchini
- Two cups spinach, roughly chopped
- Half cup bamboo shoots, canned & strained
- Two tbsp garlic-infused olive oil (green tops only)
- Two tbsp tamari sauce (low-sodium)
- Two tbsp lemon juice
- Half tsp ginger powder
- Quarter tsp black pepper
- Quarter tsp salt

Directions:

1. Heat one tbsp garlic-infused olive oil in your big skillet on moderate temp. Add diced turkey, then cook within 5-7 mins, mixing often. Put aside.
2. In your same skillet, heat another tbsp garlic-infused olive oil. Add bell pepper plus zucchini, then cook within 3 to 4 mins till vegetables start to soften.
3. Add spinach and bamboo shoots, mixing till spinach is wilted.
4. Add cooked turkey to your skillet. Mix in tamari sauce, lemon juice, ginger powder, black pepper, plus salt. Cook within two minutes till blended. Serve.

Nutritional Values (per serving): *Calories: 280; Carbs: 12g; Fat: 12g; Protein: 30g; Fiber: 3g*

NOTES

_____

_____

34. Roasted Garlic and Herb Pork Tenderloin

Preparation time: 15 minutes
Cooking time: 24 minutes
Servings: 4

Ingredients:

- ☐ One (one & half pounds) pork tenderloin
- ☐ Two tbsp garlic-infused olive oil
- ☐ One tbsp chopped each rosemary, thyme & oregano
- ☐ One tsp salt
- ☐ Half tsp ground black pepper
- ☐ Two tbsp unsalted butter

Directions:

1. Warm up your oven to 400°F.
2. In your small container, mix garlic-infused olive oil, rosemary, thyme, oregano, salt, plus black pepper.
3. Put pork tenderloin in your baking dish, then rub herb mixture all over meat. Warm up your big oven-safe skillet on moderate-high temp, then dissolve butter.
4. Sear pork tenderloin within 2 mins per side till lightly browned. Move skillet to your oven, then roast within 20 mins till cooked through. Cool it down, slice, then serve.

Nutritional Values (per serving): *Calories: 300; Carbs: 1g; Fat: 18g; Protein: 30g; Fiber: 0g*

NOTES

_____

_____

_____

35. Cilantro Lime Grilled Chicken

Preparation time: 15 minutes
Cooking time: 20 minutes
Servings: 4

Ingredients:

- ☐ Four no bones & skin chicken breasts
- ☐ Quarter cup lime juice
- ☐ Half cup chopped cilantro
- ☐ One-third cup garlic-infused olive oil (make sure it's free of garlic pieces)
- ☐ One tsp ground cumin
- ☐ Half tsp smoked paprika
- ☐ Half tsp sea salt
- ☐ Quarter tsp black pepper

Directions:

1. In your big container, mix lime juice, cilantro, garlic-infused olive oil, cumin, paprika, salt, plus black pepper.
2. Add chicken breasts till coated. Marinate in your refrigerator within 1 hour. Warm up your grill to moderate-high temp. Lightly oil your grates.
3. Put marinated chicken breasts on your grill, then cook within 6 to 7 mins per side till cooked through. Remove, cool it down, then serve.

Nutritional Values (per serving): *Calories: 290; Carbs: 3g; Fat: 14g; Protein: 37g; Fiber: 1g*

NOTES

_____

_____

_____

36. Lemon Roasted Green Beans

Preparation time: 10 minutes
Cooking time: 18 minutes
Servings: 4

Ingredients:

- [ ] One-pound green beans, ends trimmed
- [ ] Two tbsp garlic-infused olive oil
- [ ] Zest of one lemon
- [ ] One tbsp lemon juice
- [ ] Half a tsp salt
- [ ] Quarter tsp black pepper, ground

Directions:

1. Warm up your oven to 425°F.
2. In your big container, mix green beans, garlic-infused olive oil, zest, lemon juice, salt, plus black pepper. Transfer seasoned green beans to your big baking sheet.
3. Roast within 15-18 mins till slightly browned, shaking your basket once. Serve.

Nutritional Values (per serving): *Calories 134; Carbs 14g; Fat 9g; Protein 4g; Fiber 6g*

NOTES

_____

_____

_____

37. Baked Cod with Herbs and Lemon

Preparation time: 15 minutes
Cooking time: 20 minutes
Servings: 4

Ingredients:

- ☐ Four (six-oz) cod fillets
- ☐ One tbsp chopped each parsley, chives & dill
- ☐ One tsp grated lemon zest
- ☐ One tbsp lemon juice
- ☐ Two tbsp extra virgin olive oil
- ☐ Quarter tsp each sea salt & ground black pepper

Directions:

1. Warm up your oven to 400°F.
2. In your small container, mix parsley, chives, dill, zest, and lemon juice.
3. Lay cod fillets on your lined baking sheet, then brush each fillet with half tbsp of olive oil. Flavor fillets using salt plus pepper.
4. Spoon herb and lemon mixture atop each fillet. Drizzle remaining one tbsp olive oil on the fillets. Bake within 18-20 mins till cod flakes easily. Serve.

Nutritional Values (per serving): *Calories: 210; Carbs: 1g; Fat: 9g; Protein: 30g; Fiber: 0g*

NOTES

_____

_____

_____

38. Garlic and Herb Roasted Pork Chops

Preparation time: 15 minutes
Cooking time: 25 minutes
Servings: 4

Ingredients:

- ☐ Four no bones pork chops, about one-inch thick
- ☐ Two tbsp of garlic-infused olive oil (made with garlic cloves discarded)
- ☐ One tbsp chopped each rosemary & thyme
- ☐ Half tsp each ground black pepper & sea salt

Directions:

1. Warm up your oven to 400°F.
2. In your small container, mix garlic-infused olive oil, rosemary, thyme, salt, plus pepper.
3. Put pork chops in your lined baking dish. Rub herb mixture evenly onto each pork chop.
4. Bake within 20-25 mins, flipping once till cooked through. Serve.

Nutritional Values (per serving): *Calories: 297; Carbs: 1g; Fat: 21g; Protein: 25g; Fiber: 0g*

NOTES

39. Butternut Squash and Sage Soup

Preparation time: 15 minutes
Cooking time: 45 minutes
Servings: 4

Ingredients:

- One medium butternut squash, peeled, deseeded, & sliced into cubes
- Two tbsp olive oil
- One tsp garlic-infused olive oil
- Three cups chicken broth, low-sodium
- Ten fresh sage leaves, chopped finely
- One-fourth tsp ground black pepper
- One-fourth tsp sea salt

Directions:

1. Warm up your oven to 400°F.
2. In your big container, toss cubed butternut squash and olive oil, then spread on your lined baking sheet.
3. Roast squash within 25 to 30 mins till slightly golden brown. Remove, then cool it down.
4. In your big saucepan on moderate temp, add garlic-infused olive oil, then warm it up. Add roasted butternut squash, plus broth. Let it boil.
5. Add sage leaves, black pepper, plus sea salt, then simmer within 15 mins. Blend the soup using your immersion blender till smooth. Serve hot.

Nutritional Values (per serving): *Calories: 275; Carbs: 45g; Fat: 10g; Protein: 6g; Fiber: 7g*

NOTES

_____

_____

_____

40. Grilled Lemon Herb Chicken Skewers

Preparation time: 15 minutes
Cooking time: 10 minutes
Servings: 4

Ingredients:

- [ ] One & half pounds no bones & skin chicken breasts, cubes
- [ ] Two medium-sized lemons, juiced
- [ ] Three tbsp garlic-infused olive oil (use only the oil)
- [ ] One tbsp chopped each parsley, basil & oregano
- [ ] One tsp salt
- [ ] Half-tsp black pepper

Directions:

1. In your big container, mix lemon juice, garlic-infused olive oil, parsley, basil, oregano, salt, plus pepper.
2. Add cubed chicken, then toss till fully coated. Marinate within 30 mins in your refrigerator. Warm up your grill to moderate-high temp.
3. Thread marinated chicken onto your metal skewers. Put skewers on your grill, then cook within 5 mins on each side till chicken is fully cooked through.

Nutritional Values (per serving): *Calories: 265; Carbs: 3g; Fat: 11g; Protein: 37g; Fiber: 0g*

NOTES

_____

_____

_____

41. Rosemary and Garlic Roasted Lamb Chops

Preparation time: 10 minutes
Cooking time: 20 minutes
Servings: 4

Ingredients:

- ☐ Eight lamb chops
- ☐ Two tbsp garlic-infused olive oil
- ☐ Two tbsp chopped fresh rosemary
- ☐ Half tsp black pepper, ground
- ☐ Half tsp sea salt
- ☐ One tbsp white wine vinegar

Directions:

1. Warm up your oven to 400°F.
2. In your small container, mix garlic-infused olive oil, rosemary, pepper, sea salt, plus white wine vinegar. Put lamb chops on your lined baking sheet.
3. Rub rosemary-garlic mixture evenly onto lamb chops. Roast the lamb chops within 15 to 20 mins till cooked through. Remove, cool it down, then serve.

Nutritional Values (per serving): *Calories: 290; Carbs: 1g; Fat: 19g; Protein: 25g; Fiber: 1g*

NOTES

_____

_____

_____

42. Cumin-Spiced Roasted Carrots

Preparation time: 10 minutes
Cooking time: 25 minutes
Servings: 4

Ingredients:

- ☐ Eight medium carrots, peeled & halved lengthwise
- ☐ Two tbsp garlic-infused olive oil (make sure it's low-FODMAP)
- ☐ One & half tsp cumin, ground
- ☐ Half tsp paprika
- ☐ Quarter tsp each turmeric & ground coriander
- ☐ Salt & ground black pepper, as required

Directions:

1. Warm up your oven to 425°F.
2. In your big container, whisk garlic-infused olive oil, cumin, paprika, turmeric, coriander, salt, plus black pepper. Add carrots, then toss gently.
3. Lay out seasoned carrots on your lined baking sheet. Roast carrots within 25 mins till tender, turning them once. Serve.

Nutritional Values (per serving): *Calories: 130; Carbs: 14g; Fat: 8g; Protein: 2g ; Fiber: 4g*

NOTES

_____

_____

_____

43. Turkey Burgers with Tzatziki Sauce

Preparation time: 20 minutes
Cooking time: 15 minutes
Servings: 4

Ingredients:

- ☐ One & quarter pounds ground turkey
- ☐ One tbsp chopped each oregano & parsley
- ☐ One tsp garlic-infused olive oil
- ☐ Half tsp salt
- ☐ Quarter tsp ground black pepper
- ☐ Four leaves of lettuce (for serving)

For the Tzatziki Sauce:

- ☐ Half cup lactose-free Greek yogurt
- ☐ Two tbsp chopped fresh dill
- ☐ Two tbsp lemon juice
- ☐ Half cup grated & strained cucumber
- ☐ Quarter tsp salt

Directions:

1. In your big bowl, mix ground turkey, oregano, parsley, garlic-infused olive oil, salt, plus black pepper. Form into four patties.
2. Warm up your grill to moderate-high temp. Cook patties within 6 to 7 mins per side till cooked through. Remove, then cool it down.
3. Meanwhile, prepare the tzatziki sauce. Mix Greek yogurt, dill, lemon juice, grated cucumber, and salt in your small container.
4. To serve, place each burger on a lettuce leaf, then topped with tzatziki sauce.

Nutritional Values (per serving): *Calories: 345; Carbs: 8g; Fat: 20g; Protein: 32g; Fiber: 1g*

NOTES

---

44. Ginger and Turmeric Baked Chicken Thighs

Preparation time: 15 minutes
Cooking time: 45 minutes
Servings: 4

Ingredients:

- ☐ Four bone-in, skin-on chicken thighs
- ☐ Two tbsp extra-virgin olive oil
- ☐ One tsp ground each ginger & turmeric
- ☐ Half tsp each ground black pepper & sea salt
- ☐ Two medium-sized carrots, peeled & sliced into thin strips
- ☐ One cup diced zucchini

Directions:

1. Warm up your oven to 375°F.
2. In your small container, mix ginger, turmeric, black pepper, plus sea salt. Rub chicken thighs using olive oil, then coat them with spice mixture.
3. Put seasoned chicken thighs on your lined baking tray lined. Scatter carrots and zucchini around chicken thighs. Bake within 45 mins till cooked through. Serve.

Nutritional Values (per serving): *Calories: 285; Carbs: 6g; Fat: 18g; Protein: 23g; Fiber: 2g*

NOTES

_____

_____

_____

45. Lemon Garlic Roasted Brussels Sprouts

Preparation time: 15 minutes
Cooking time: 25 minutes
Servings: 4

Ingredients:

- ☐ One pound Brussels sprouts, halved
- ☐ Two tbsp garlic-infused olive oil
- ☐ One tbsp lemon juice
- ☐ One tsp lemon zest
- ☐ Half tsp sea salt
- ☐ Quarter tsp black pepper, ground

Directions:

1. Warm up your oven to 400°F.
2. In your big container, mix Brussels sprouts, garlic-infused olive oil, juice, and zest.
3. Spread Brussels sprouts onto your baking sheet. Sprinkle using sea salt plus black pepper.
4. Roast within 25 mins till Brussels sprouts are tender. Serve.

Nutritional Values (per serving): *Calories: 110; Carbs: 10g; Fat: 7g; Protein: 4g; Fiber: 4g*

NOTES

_____

_____

_____

46. Moroccan-Spiced Roasted Cauliflower

Preparation time: 15 minutes
Cooking time: 25 minutes
Servings: 4

Ingredients:

- [ ] One big head cauliflower, florets
- [ ] Two tbsp garlic-infused olive oil
- [ ] Half tsp each cumin, paprika, ground coriander & ground ginger
- [ ] Quarter tsp each ground cinnamon & turmeric
- [ ] Salt & ground black pepper, as required

Directions:

1. Warm up your oven to 425°F.
2. In your small container, mix cumin, paprika, coriander, ginger, cinnamon, and turmeric.
3. Put cauliflower florets in your big container, then drizzle with garlic-infused olive oil. Mix well.
4. Add mixed spices to your cauliflower florets, then toss well. Flavor it using salt plus black pepper.
5. Spread seasoned cauliflower florets on your lined baking sheet. Roast within 25 mins till cauliflower is slightly crispy. Serve.

Nutritional Values (per serving): *Calories: 137; Carbs: 12g; Fat: 9g; Protein: 5g; Fiber: 5g*

NOTES

_____

_____

_____

47. Sesame-Ginger Grilled Salmon

Preparation time: 15 minutes
Cooking time: 10 minutes
Servings: 4

Ingredients:

- ☐ Four (six-oz) salmon fillets
- ☐ One tbsp sesame oil
- ☐ One tbsp grated fresh ginger
- ☐ Two tbsp soy sauce, low-sodium (gluten-free if necessary)
- ☐ One tbsp each rice vinegar & lemon juice
- ☐ Two tsp pure maple syrup
- ☐ Half tsp ground black pepper

Directions:

1. In your small container, whisk sesame oil, grated ginger, soy sauce, vinegar, lemon juice, maple syrup, and black pepper.
2. Put salmon fillets in your shallow container, then pour marinade on them. Cover, then refrigerate within 30 mins.
3. Warm up your grill to moderate-high temp. Lightly oil your grates. Put marinated fillets on your grill. Cook salmon within 4 to 5 mins per side till it flakes easily. Serve.

__Nutritional Values (per serving):__ Calories: 348; Carbs: 4g; Fat: 20g; Protein: 35g; Fiber: 0g

NOTES

_____

_____

_____

48. Basil Pesto Grilled Chicken

Preparation time: 15 minutes
Cooking time: 16 minutes
Servings: 4

Ingredients:

- ☐ Four no bones & skin chicken breasts
- ☐ One cup basil leaves, fresh
- ☐ One-third cup Parmesan cheese, grated
- ☐ One-third cup garlic-infused olive oil (strained to remove solids)
- ☐ One-fourth cup pine nuts, lightly toasted
- ☐ One tbsp lemon juice
- ☐ Salt & pepper, as required

Directions:

1. Mix basil leaves, Parmesan cheese, toasted pine nuts, and juice in your food processor. Pulse till coarsely chopped.
2. Slowly drizzle in garlic-infused olive oil while pulsing. Flavor it using salt plus pepper.
3. Put chicken breasts in your shallow container, then flavor it using plus and pepper. Spread pesto on each chicken breast.
4. Warm up your grill on moderate-high temp. Put pesto-coated chicken breasts on your grill, then cook within 6-8 mins per side till cooked through. Remove, cool it down, then serve.

Nutritional Values (per serving): *Calories: 425; Carbs: 4g; Fat: 28g; Protein: 38g; Fiber: 1g*

NOTES

_____

_____

_____

49. Cumin and Paprika Roasted Pork Tenderloin

Preparation time: 10 minutes
Cooking time: 25 minutes
Servings: 4

Ingredients:

- ☐ One pork tenderloin (one & quarter pounds), pat dried
- ☐ Two tbsp olive oil, extra virgin
- ☐ One tbsp cumin, ground
- ☐ One tbsp smoked paprika
- ☐ Half tsp salt
- ☐ Quarter tsp black pepper

Directions:

1. Warm up your oven to 400°F.
2. In your small container, mix cumin, paprika, salt, plus black pepper. Rub pork tenderloin with one tbsp olive oil. Sprinkle spice mixture on the tenderloin, then rub it till coated.
3. Warm up remaining olive oil in your oven-safe skillet on moderate-high temp. Sear tenderloin within 2 mins per side till browned.
4. Move skillet your oven, then roast within 20-25 mins till cooked through. Remove, cool it down, slice, then serve.

Nutritional Values (per serving): *Calories: 260; Carbs: 2g; Fat: 15g; Protein: 29g; Fiber: 1g*

NOTES

_____

_____

_____

50. Shrimp and Vegetable Stir-Fry

Preparation time: 15 minutes
Cooking time: 10 minutes
Servings: 4

Ingredients:

- [ ] One pound shrimp, peeled & cleaned
- [ ] One cup chopped each green & red bell pepper
- [ ] One-half cup thinly sliced carrots
- [ ] One-fourth cup chopped green onion tops (green part only)
- [ ] Two tbsp garlic-infused oil, divided
- [ ] One tbsp fresh grated ginger
- [ ] Two tbsp Tamari soy sauce, gluten-free
- [ ] Two tbsp rice vinegar
- [ ] One tbsp brown sugar replacement (e.g. Swerve Brown)
- [ ] Salt & black pepper, as required

Directions:

1. In your small container, whisk Tamari soy sauce, vinegar, and brown sugar. Put aside.
2. Warm up one tbsp garlic-infused oil in your big skillet on moderate-high temp. Add shrimp, then cook within 3-4 mins till pink. Put aside.
3. In your same skillet, warm up remaining garlic-infused oil. Add sliced carrots, then cook within 2 mins till slightly softened. Add bell peppers, then cook within 2 mins.
4. Add green onion tops and ginger, then cook within one min. Add cooked shrimp, then pour sauce mixture. Mix well.
5. Cook within 2-minute till sauce has thickened slightly. Flavor it using salt plus black pepper. Serve.

Nutritional Values (per serving): *Calories: 230; Carbs: 12g; Fat: 9g; Protein: 25g; Fiber: 2g*

NOTES

_____

_____

_____

51. Herb-Marinated Grilled Steak

Preparation time: 10 minutes + marinating time
Cooking time: 10 minutes
Servings: 4

Ingredients:

- ☐ Two pounds sirloin steak
- ☐ One tbsp garlic-infused olive oil
- ☐ One tbsp balsamic vinegar
- ☐ One tbsp lemon juice
- ☐ Two tsp dried each oregano, thyme & rosemary
- ☐ Half tsp each salt & ground black pepper

Directions:

1. In your small container, whisk garlic-infused olive oil, vinegar, juice, oregano, thyme, rosemary, salt, plus pepper.
2. Put sirloin steak in your big zip-top bag, then pour marinade. Seal, then marinate in your refrigerator within 2 hours, turning often.
3. Warm up your grill to moderate-high temp.
4. Put marinated steak on your grill, then cook within five mins per side for medium-rare to medium doneness. Remove, cool it down, slice, then serve.

Nutritional Values (per serving): *Calories: 390; Carbs: 3g; Fat: 22g; Protein: 45g; Fiber: 1g*

NOTES

_____

_____

_____

52. Turmeric-Roasted Cauliflower Rice

Preparation time: 10 minutes
Cooking time: 25 minutes
Servings: 4

Ingredients:

- [ ] One big head cauliflower, grated
- [ ] Two tbsp olive oil
- [ ] One tsp ground turmeric
- [ ] One tbsp lemon juice
- [ ] Salt & pepper, as required

Directions:

1. Warm up your oven to 400°F. Put grated cauliflower in your big container.
2. In your small container, whisk olive oil, turmeric, lemon juice, salt, plus pepper. Drizzle turmeric mixture on cauliflower rice, then toss well.
3. Spread seasoned cauliflower onto your lined baking sheet. Roast within 25 mins till golden brown, mixing often. Serve.

Nutritional Values (per serving): *Calories: 114; Carbs: 9g; Fat: 8g; Protein: 3g; Fiber: 4g*

NOTES

_____

_____

_____

53. Garlic and Herb Roasted Turkey Legs

Preparation time: 20 minutes
Cooking time: 1 hour & 30 minutes
Servings: 4

Ingredients:

- [ ] Four medium-sized turkey legs
- [ ] One tbsp garlic-infused olive oil
- [ ] One tbsp chopped each thyme & rosemary
- [ ] Half tsp salt
- [ ] Half tsp black pepper, ground
- [ ] Quarter cup chopped scallions (green tops only)
- [ ] Two tbsp butter, melted

Directions:

1. Warm up your oven to 375°F.
2. In your small container, mix garlic-infused olive oil, thyme, rosemary, salt, plus black pepper. Rub turkey legs with herb mixture.
3. Put turkey legs on your roasting tray, then sprinkle scallions on top. Pour butter evenly across turkey legs.
4. Bake within1 hour and 30 mins till cooked through. Remove, cool it down, then serve.

Nutritional Values (per serving): *Calories: 475; Carbs: 2g; Fat: 24g; Protein: 62g; Fiber: 1g*

NOTES

_____

_____

_____

54. Rosemary and Lemon Grilled Lamb Chops

Preparation time: 15 minutes + marinating time
Cooking time: 10 minutes
Servings: 4

Ingredients:

- ☐ Eight lamb chops
- ☐ Two tbsp chopped rosemary
- ☐ One large lemon, zested & juiced
- ☐ Three tbsp garlic-infused olive oil
- ☐ One tbsp sea salt
- ☐ Half tsp black pepper, ground

Directions:

1. In your small container, mix rosemary, zest, lemon juice, garlic-infused olive oil, sea salt, plus black pepper.
2. Put lamb chops in your shallow container, then pour marinade. Cover, then marinate within 30 mins in your refrigerator.
3. Warm up your grill to moderate-high temp. Put marinated lamb chops on your grill, then cook within 4-5 mins on each side till cooked through. Remove, cool it down, then serve.

Nutritional Values (per serving): *Calories: 350; Carbs: 2g; Fat: 24g; Protein: 30g; Fiber: 1g*

NOTES

_____

_____

_____

55. Cilantro Lime Shrimp and Avocado Salad

Preparation time: 20 minutes
Cooking time: 5 minutes
Servings: 4

Ingredients:

- One-pound medium shrimp, peeled & cleaned
- One medium Hass avocado, diced
- Quarter cup chopped cilantro
- Two tbsp each extra virgin olive oil & lime juice
- Half tsp each cumin, paprika & garlic-infused olive oil
- Salt & pepper, as required
- Four cups of mixed greens (e.g., spinach, arugula)

Directions:

1. In your big container, mix oil, lime juice, garlic-infused olive oil, cumin, paprika, salt, plus pepper. Add shrimp, then toss well. Marinate within 10 mins.
2. Warm up your big non-stick skillet on moderate-high temp. Add marinated shrimp, then cook within 2 to 3 mins per side till they turn pink.
3. In your big serving container, combine mixed greens, avocado and cilantro. Top it with cooked shrimp. Serve.

Nutritional Values (per serving): *Calories: 300; Carbs: 10g; Fat: 18g; Protein: 26g; Fiber: 5g*

NOTES

_____

_____

_____

56. Roasted Butternut Squash and Brussels Sprouts

Preparation time: 15 minutes
Cooking time: 30 minutes
Servings: 4

Ingredients:

- ☐ One small butternut squash, peeled, seeded, & sliced into cubes
- ☐ One pound Brussels sprouts, trimmed & halved
- ☐ Two tbsp garlic-infused olive oil (discard any garlic pieces)
- ☐ One tsp dried each thyme & rosemary
- ☐ Salt & pepper, as required
- ☐ Two tbsp lemon juice

Directions:

1. Warm up your oven to 400°F.
2. In your big bowl, mix butternut squash plus Brussels sprouts.
3. Drizzle garlic-infused olive oil, then sprinkle with thyme, rosemary, salt, plus pepper. Toss well. Spread vegetables on your lined baking sheet.
4. Roast within 25-30 mins till vegetables are tender, mixing them once. Remove, then drizzle with lemon juice. Serve.

Nutritional Values (per serving): *Calories: 168; Carbs: 27g; Fat: 7g; Protein: 4g; Fiber: 6g*

NOTES

_____

_____

_____

57. Greek Lemon Chicken Soup

Preparation time: 15 minutes
Cooking time: 30 minutes
Servings: 4

Ingredients:

- ☐ One-pound no bones & skin chicken breasts, diced
- ☐ Two tbsp olive oil
- ☐ Quarter cup lemon juice
- ☐ Six cups low-sodium chicken broth
- ☐ One cup water
- ☐ One-half cup white rice (uncooked)
- ☐ One cup baby spinach, chopped
- ☐ Two big eggs
- ☐ Salt & pepper, as required

Directions:

1. Warm up your big pot on moderate-high temp. Add olive oil plus diced chicken breasts.
2. Cook chicken within 5 mins till browned. Flavor it using salt plus pepper. Add broth, water, and uncooked rice.
3. Let it boil, adjust to a simmer, then cover. Simmer within 20 mins till rice is cooked through. Mix in chopped baby spinach, then cook within 2-3 mins till wilted.
4. In your separate container, whisk eggs plus lemon juice till smooth. Slowly ladle 1 cup hot broth into your egg-lemon mixture while whisking to temper eggs.
5. Pour tempered egg-lemon mixture into your soup pot while mixing. Simmer within 2 mins to thicken the soup slightly. Serve.

Nutritional Values (per serving): *Calories: 325; Carbs: 23g; Fat: 14g; Protein: 30g; Fiber: 1g*

NOTES

_____

_____

58. Baked Ginger Soy Salmon

Preparation time: 15 minutes
Cooking time: 20 minutes
Servings: 4

Ingredients:

- ☐ Four (six-oz) salmon fillets
- ☐ Two tbsp soy sauce, low-sodium
- ☐ One tbsp freshly grated ginger
- ☐ One tbsp garlic-infused olive oil
- ☐ Half tsp sesame oil
- ☐ Two green onion tops, thinly sliced (green portions only)
- ☐ One tbsp chopped cilantro leaves
- ☐ Quarter tsp ground black pepper
- ☐ Salt, as required

Directions:

1. Warm up your oven to 400°F.
2. In your small container, mix soy sauce, ginger, garlic-infused olive oil, sesame oil, plus ground black pepper
3. Put salmon fillets on your baking sheet. Brush each fillet with ginger soy mixture. Sprinkle salt on each salmon fillet.
4. Bake salmon within12-15 mins till is fish flakes easily. Remove, then sprinkle with green onion tops and cilantro.

Nutritional Values (per serving): *Calories: 350; Carbs: 3g; Fat: 22g; Protein: 34g; Fiber: 0g*

NOTES

_____

_____

_____

59. Grilled Tandoori Chicken with Mint Chutney

Preparation time: 20 minutes
Cooking time: 25 minutes
Servings: 4

Ingredients:

- ☐ One & half pounds no bones & skin chicken thighs
- ☐ One tbsp garlic-infused oil
- ☐ One tbsp grated ginger
- ☐ Two tbsp lactose-free Greek yogurt
- ☐ One tbsp lemon juice
- ☐ One tsp ground cumin
- ☐ Half tsp each paprika, ground coriander & turmeric
- ☐ Quarter tsp each cayenne pepper & salt

For the Mint Chutney:

- ☐ Half cup chopped each mint & cilantro leaves
- ☐ Two tbsp garlic-infused oil
- ☐ One tbsp finely chopped green onion tops (only the green part)
- ☐ One tbsp lemon juice
- ☐ Salt & pepper, as required

Directions:

1. In your container, mix garlic-infused oil, ginger, Greek yogurt, lemon juice, cumin, paprika, coriander, turmeric, cayenne pepper, plus salt.
2. Add chicken thighs, then mix well. Cover, then refrigerate within 2 hours. Warm up your grill to moderate-high temp. Thread chicken thighs onto skewers.
3. Grill chicken within 10 to 12 mins on each side till fully cooked.
4. For the mint chutney, in your food processor, add mint, cilantro, garlic-infused oil, green onion tops, lemon juice, salt plus pepper. Blend till smooth.
5. Serve grilled tandoori chicken with mint chutney on the side.

Nutritional Values (per serving): *Calories: 350; Carbs: 7g; Fat: 20g; Protein: 35g; Fiber: 2g*

NOTES

_____

_____

60. Lemon Herb Grilled Shrimp

Preparation time: 10 minutes
Cooking time: 6 minutes
Servings: 4

Ingredients:

- [ ] One-pound large shrimp, peeled & cleaned
- [ ] Three tbsp garlic-infused olive oil
- [ ] Two tbsp chopped fresh parsley
- [ ] One tbsp chopped each cilantro & basil
- [ ] One tbsp lemon juice
- [ ] One tsp lemon zest
- [ ] Half tsp salt
- [ ] Quarter tsp black pepper, ground

Directions:

1. In your medium container, whisk garlic-infused olive oil, parsley, cilantro, basil, lemon juice, zest, salt, plus black pepper.
2. Add shrimp, then mix well till coated. Marinate within 15-20 mins in your refrigerator.
3. Warm up grill to moderate-high temp. Lightly oil your grates. Thread shrimp onto skewers.
4. Grill shrimp within 2-3 mins per side till pink. Serve.

Nutritional Values (per serving): *Calories: 190; Carbs: 1g; Fat: 11g; Protein: 21g; Fiber: 0g*

NOTES

_____
_____
_____

Encouraging Children to Embrace Healthy Eating Habits

Children are naturally attracted to vibrant colors, creative shapes, and delicious flavors. As parents or guardians, it is essential to encourage them to embrace healthy eating habits, especially when following the SIBO Diet. By doing so, not only can we ensure their growth and development but also instill positive lifelong eating habits that contribute to their overall well-being.

Healthy eating habits are crucial for children diagnosed with SIBO or exhibiting symptoms of the condition. The SIBO diet focuses on reducing the fermentable carbohydrates in an individual's diet that feed the present bacteria in their small intestine. Consequently, this section will provide insightful tips on how to encourage children to adopt wholesome SIBO diets.

1. Make It Fun and Creative: Children adore fun and creativity. When it comes to food preparation, it is the ideal opportunity to make dishes visually appealing and enticing. Transforming a simple meal into a piece of art will engage your child's curiosity and make them more eager to try out new, healthy foods. Use cookie cutters for sandwich shapes, create funny faces using vegetable cutouts or even plan a theme-based meal based on their favorite cartoon characters. The key is to think outside the box and captivate their imagination while introducing nutritious meal components.

2. Engage Them in Planning and Preparing Meals: Children are more likely to eat healthier if they are involved in planning and preparing meals. Encourage your child to participate in choosing recipes, grocery shopping, and cooking new meals alongside you in the kitchen. Assign specific age-appropriate tasks such as washing fruits and vegetables, stirring ingredients, or plating dishes beautifully under your guidance. This involvement allows them to take ownership of their meals while learning about nutritious foods directly fostering an appreciation for healthy eating habits.

3. Educate Them About SIBO Diet: Educating children about the SIBO diet and its importance is vital to encourage them to embrace healthy food choices. Sit down with your child and explain how certain foods may hinder their gut health, using simple terms and illustrations. Instead of forcing them to consume specific foods, educate them about the benefits of a balanced meal rich in proteins, vitamins, and low in fermentable carbohydrates. This knowledge will empower them to make informed decisions about their dietary choices in the long run.

4. Establish Routines and Be Consistent: Consistency plays a significant role in forming any habit. Establish a consistent routine for your child's meal timings, portion sizes, and snacking habits. Make sure that the whole family follows the same routine to create a common understanding and support system, especially if someone else in your household has SIBO or a digestive disorder. This approach will also make it easier for your child to accept alterations in their dietary lifestyle.

5. Offer Healthy Snacks and Treats: Children love snacks, but most commonly available options are unhealthy and contain high amounts of sugar or processed ingredients. Embrace creative ways to present fruits, nuts, seeds, or homemade SIBO-friendly treats as eye-catching snack options rather than chips or candies. Besides, serve healthier treat alternatives like smoothie bowls or SIBO-friendly granola bars on special occasions. By doing so, you'll teach children that there are nutritious choices available that taste just as great.

6. Be Patient and Positive: Changing eating habits is challenging for everyone – adults and children alike. Approach this process with patience as children have individual preferences that could take time to adapt to the SIBO diet requirements. Praise small successes while maintaining positivity throughout the transition phase. Children learn best from observing adult behavior; hence your positive attitude towards healthy diets will significantly impact their motivation.

Helping children adopt healthy eating habits within a SIBO diet requires a combination of creativity, consistency, education, involvement, and patience. By incorporating these tips into daily routines, your child will gradually develop a love for healthy foods that are beneficial to their overall wellness while managing the symptoms of SIBO effectively.

Balancing SIBO Diet with Family Preferences

One of the biggest hurdles for individuals with SIBO is finding a way to balance their dietary needs with the preferences and requirements of their family. This section will provide tips and suggestions for integrating a SIBO diet into everyday family life, ensuring everyone enjoys tasty and satisfying meals together.

1. Communication is key: The first step in managing the complexity of a SIBO diet within a family is open communication. It's important to discuss your dietary restrictions and needs with your family members to ensure they understand why certain foods must be avoided. Education about SIBO and its impacts on your health can help foster understanding and support from your loved ones.

2. Get creative with substitutions: The SIBO diet may require some adjustments when it comes to meal planning and recipes but think of this as an opportunity to get creative in the kitchen. Experiment with alternative ingredients like herbs and spices that are approved for the SIBO diet list, such as basil, oregano, thyme, or turmeric. You can also try using almond flour or coconut flour instead of wheat-based products for those following a low FODMAP regimen.

3. Find common ground: When planning meals, focus on finding dishes that satisfy both your SIBO dietary needs and the taste preferences of your family members. Many traditional dishes can be easily adapted to suit a SIBO diet by making simple ingredient substitutions or tweaks while still maintaining the overall flavor profile of the dish.

4. Cook in batches: One practical way to accommodate different dietary needs within a household is by batch cooking meals that can be portioned out and customized for each family member. For example, you might prepare your big pot of chili where you can add beans or other high-FODMAP ingredients to individual portions for those without SIBO restrictions.

5. Family-style dining: Another option for balancing a SIBO diet with family preferences is to offer a variety of dishes that are served family-style. This way, each family member can pick and choose which dishes they want to eat from, ensuring everyone has an enjoyable meal while still respecting your dietary needs.

6. Encourage everyone to try new foods: When introducing new SIBO-friendly recipes, encourage your entire family to try these dishes. In doing so, you will not only expose them to new flavors and textures but also demonstrate that a SIBO diet can be diverse and delicious.

7. Enlist family members in meal planning and preparation: Involving your family in the meal planning process can help bridge the gap between your SIBO restrictions and their preferences. By giving them a say in the foods that are on the menu, they may be more willing to try new recipes or make adjustments to suit your dietary needs.

8. Keep snacks accessible: To accommodate various food preferences and dietary restrictions within a household, it's important to keep a variety of SIBO-approved snacks on hand. Stock up on items like rice cakes, almond butter, carrots, celery or homemade trail mix so you have something satisfying to snack on when hunger strikes.

9. Seek support: Connecting with others living with SIBO can provide valuable insights and support as you navigate balancing your diet with family preferences. Look for online forums, support groups or community events where you can share experiences and learn from others facing similar challenges.

10. Celebrate successes: As you find ways to successfully balance a SIBO diet with your family's preferences, remember to celebrate your achievements. Enjoy shared meals not only as nourishment but also as an opportunity for connection and bonding with your loved ones.

Managing a SIBO diet alongside family preferences can be a delicate balance. With effective communication, creativity, flexibility, and support, it's possible to maintain an enjoyable and satisfying dining experience for both you and your loved ones. Implementing the tips outlined above can help to enhance your family's understanding while ensuring that both your SIBO dietary needs and their preferences are met.

CHAPTER 10:
SUSTAINING YOUR
SIBO SUCCESS

Managing SIBO and preventing its recurrence can be challenging, but it's crucial for your long-term health and well-being. This article will explore strategies for long-term SIBO management, monitoring and tracking symptoms, and embracing a lifetime of gut-friendly habits.

Strategies for Long-term SIBO Management

1. Diet Modification: A low-FODMAP diet has been proven to be effective in reducing symptoms associated with SIBO. This diet involves eliminating foods that are high in fermentable sugars that can cause gas, bloating, and discomfort. Gradually reintroduce these foods as your symptoms improve to determine which ones you tolerate well.

2. Probiotics: Using probiotics is beneficial for maintaining the proper balance of good bacteria in the gut. Choose a high-quality probiotic supplement with a variety of strains specifically designed to support gut health and prevent SIBO recurrence.

3. Stress Management: Stress can impact your gut health and contribute to the development of SIBO. Incorporate stress-relieving activities like yoga, meditation, or deep breathing exercises into your daily routine to support both mental and physical well-being.

4. Regular Exercise: Physical activity supports healthy digestion by promoting bowel movement and encouraging the growth of good gut bacteria. Make it a point to engage in regular exercise that you enjoy to support long-term SIBO management.

Monitoring and Tracking Symptoms

1. Keep a Food Diary: Recording what you eat daily can help you notice patterns between specific foods and SIBO symptoms like bloating or diarrhea. Use this information to make adjustments to your diet accordingly.

2. Develop a Symptom-Tracking System: Track your symptoms daily using either a notebook or an app to better understand your body's response to various triggers. This information will be invaluable for managing your condition effectively.

3. Check-In with a Healthcare Professional: Schedule regular appointments with your healthcare provider to discuss progress, address symptoms, and adjust treatment plans accordingly. Open communication with your doctor is crucial for long-term success in managing SIBO.

4. Stay Informed: Research about SIBO is constantly advancing, so keep yourself updated on the latest findings and news about the condition. Join online support groups or forums to connect with others experiencing similar challenges.

Embracing a Lifetime of Gut-friendly Habits

1. Prioritize Gut Health: Make choices that promote gut health in every aspect of your life— from the food you eat to the activities you participate in. Recognize the critical role that gut health plays in your overall wellness.

2. Develop Sustainable Habits: It's essential to maintain long-term habits that promote gut health rather than resorting to short-term fixes that could lead to recurrence of SIBO.

3. Maintain Balance: Eat a variety of foods that provide the necessary nutrients for good gut health without causing SIBO flare-ups. Avoid binge eating or restrictive diets that can disrupt the balance of your gut microbiome.

4. Be Patient and Persistent: SIBO management can be an ongoing process, and setbacks may occur along the way. Focus on progress rather than perfection, and remember that consistency in practicing healthy habits is crucial for long-term success.

Effectively managing SIBO requires adopting long-term strategies that support gut health, monitoring and tracking symptoms closely, and embracing a lifestyle centered around gut-friendly habits. By adhering to these principles, you'll be better equipped to sustain your SIBO success and enjoy improved overall well-being.

CONCLUSION

Throughout this journey, we have delved deep into understanding the complexities of SIBO, its symptoms, and its impact on gut health. The guidance provided in diagnosing SIBO and consulting with healthcare professionals ensures a strong foundation for initiating the healing process.

The book's introduction to the SIBO diet and its various types empowers readers to make informed decisions for themselves. By fostering a personalized meal plan, individuals can take charge of their health and navigate the elimination phase effectively. Through the gradual reintroduction of foods within a balanced gut microbiome, readers learn to adapt to a new way of eating that supports their recovery.

Meal planning and preparation techniques, along with tips for dining out and traveling on the SIBO diet, ensure that readers can maintain their dietary choices with ease. The ability to communicate one's dietary needs effectively becomes an essential skill showcased in this book.

The crucial role of emotional eating and stress in relation to gut health is not overlooked either. Practicing mindful eating, addressing emotional triggers, and utilizing stress-reduction techniques are key strategies presented for managing SIBO effectively. The inclusion of SIBO-friendly family meals eases the transition into healthier eating habits for the whole family while also accommodating dietary restrictions.

Lastly, sustaining long-term SIBO success is emphasized as an ongoing process. By integrating monitoring, symptom tracking, and embracing gut-friendly habits as a new way of life; readers are well-equipped to confront any future challenges linked to their gut health.

Through comprehensive advice and practical tips covering every aspect of living with SIBO, this book provides a roadmap for those navigating this journey - ultimately offering hope and inspiration towards reclaiming one's health and wellbeing.